THE FREEDOM OF THE SELF

THE BIO-EXISTENTIAL TREATMENT OF CHARACTER PROBLEMS

CRITICAL ISSUES IN PSYCHIATRY
An Educational Series for Residents and Clinicians

Series Editor: Sherwyn M. Woods, M.D., Ph.D.
University of Southern California School of Medicine
Los Angeles, California

Recent volumes in the series:

CASE STUDIES IN INSOMNIA
Edited by Peter J. Hauri, Ph.D.

CHILD AND ADULT DEVELOPMENT: A Psychoanalytic Introduction for Clinicians
Calvin A. Colarusso, M.D.

CLINICAL DISORDERS OF MEMORY
Aman U. Khan, M.D.

CONTEMPORARY PERSPECTIVES ON PSYCHOTHERAPY WITH LESBIANS AND GAY MEN
Edited by Terry S. Stein, M.D., and Carol J. Cohen, M.D.

DECIPHERING MOTIVATION IN PSYCHOTHERAPY
David M. Allen, M.D.

DIAGNOSTIC AND LABORATORY TESTING IN PSYCHIATRY
Edited by Mark S. Gold, M.D., and A. L. C. Pottash, M.D.

DRUG AND ALCOHOL ABUSE: A Clinical Guide to Diagnosis and Treatment, Third Edition
Marc A. Schuckit, M.D.

EVALUATION OF THE PSYCHIATRIC PATIENT: A Primer
Seymour L. Halleck, M.D.

THE FREEDOM OF THE SELF: The Bio-Existential Treatment of Character Problems
Eugene M. Abroms, M.D.

HANDBOOK OF BEHAVIOR THERAPY IN THE PSYCHIATRIC SETTING
Edited by Allan S. Bellack, Ph.D., and Michel Hersen, Ph.D.

NEUROPSYCHIATRIC FEATURES OF MENTAL DISORDERS
James W. Jefferson, M.D., and John R. Marshall, M.D.

RESEARCH IN PSYCHIATRY: Issues, Strategies, and Methods
Edited by L. K. George Hsu, M.D., and Michel Hersen, Ph.D.

SEXUAL LIFE: A Clinician's Guide
Stephen B. Levine, M.D.

STATES OF MIND: Configurational Analysis of Individual Psychology, Second Edition
Mardi Horowitz, M.D.

A Continuation Order Plan is available for this series. A continuation order will bring delivery of each new volume immediately upon publication. Volumes are billed only upon actual shipment. For further information please contact the publisher.

THE FREEDOM OF THE SELF

THE BIO-EXISTENTIAL TREATMENT OF CHARACTER PROBLEMS

Eugene M. Abroms, M.D.

Private Practice
Ardmore, Pennsylvania

SPRINGER SCIENCE+BUSINESS MEDIA, LLC

Library of Congress Cataloging-in-Publication Data

Abroms, Eugene M.
The freedom of the self : the bio-existential treatment of character problems / Eugene M. Abroms.
p. cm. -- (Critical issues in psychiatry)
Includes bibliographical references and index.
ISBN 978-1-4613-6255-5 ISBN 978-1-4615-2896-8 (eBook)
DOI 10.1007/978-1-4615-2896-8
1. Personality disorders--Treatment. 2. Existential psychotherapy. I. Title. II. Series.
[DNLM: 1. Behavior Therapy. 2. Psychotherapy. WM 420 A163f]
RC554.A23 1993
616.89'142--dc20
DNLM/DLC
for Library of Congress 92-48319
CIP

ISBN 978-1-4613-6255-5

Originally published by Plenum Press New York in 1993
Softcover reprint of the hardcover 1st edition 1993

To HARRIET, ADAM, RACHEL, and LISA
for filling the center of my life

Preface

My purpose in writing this book is to show how the self can be unified to expand its awareness and free its will. I shall argue that the hallmark of severe personality disorder is a dissociated self, broken up into warring subpersonalities that impede the flow of creative ideas and actions. One of these subpersonalities, an *internal saboteur*, pushes the individual into repeated acts of self-defeat. From this recognition comes a heightened appreciation of the need for unifying the self into an organized, constructive whole.

Attributing character pathology to personality dissociation, or "splitting," is not an original idea. It forms an important chapter in nineteenth-century French psychiatry, which culminated in the seminal work of Pierre Janet (1859-1947). Jung was also a strong proponent of the notion, while Fairbairn, building on the ideas of Melanie Klein, gave an illuminating account of its intrapsychic mechanisms, similar in important respects to Masterson's description of borderline pathology.

What I have added to this past work is an enhanced recognition of the close connection between splitting and unresolved traumatic grief. The clinical implications are twofold. Under the cover of other forms of pathology, patients are often found to be suffering from a split-off core depression that must be uncovered and then vigorously treated. The treatment itself is necessarily pluralistic, involving biological, behavioral, psychodynamic, social, and existential approaches.

Of these various treatment modalities, I have worked most intensively to expand the range of social and existential techniques. In my hands, sociotherapy has been developed beyond ordinary group and family therapy to yield an encompassing form of outpatient milieu therapy—extensive enough to stabilize the relationship patterns of a select group of borderline patients who tend to disrupt all their close ties. In pursuing the existential aspect of the work, I have established the importance of "holographic" intervention and beliefs, which, by integrating the previously dissociated self, leads to existential freedom, the highest goal of psychotherapy.

Becoming free depends on unifying the self both from within and from without. Internal unity yields a coherent identity with heightened self-esteem and sense of purpose. External unity involves three kinds of spiritual connection: empathic attunement with loved ones, social commitments with a higher moral purpose, and metaphysical identification with the forces of order and beauty in the universe. Individuals who have forged these unities reap the rewards of an unending psychological growth.

PLAN OF THE BOOK

The 12 chapters of this volume can be roughly divided into three main parts. The first three chapters seek to capture the spirit of a biologically oriented existential therapy (Chapter 1), to trace its past history in the archives of psychotherapy (Chapter 2), and to assemble its constituent parts from the dominant modern schools of psychiatric treatment (Chapter 3). The next four chapters set out the theoretical constructs of a bio-existential therapy, first by giving an illustrative case history (Chapter 4), then by discussing the main interpretive tools for collecting and analyzing the clinical data (Chapter 5), and then by outlining the stages of pluralistic diagnosis and treatment (Chapter 6). In the major theoretical discussion (Chapter 7), I draw together these principles to develop a grief-based account of physical and mental disorder, together with its treatment implications.

The last five chapters are devoted to various aspects of therapy technique: improving the efficacy of psychoactive medication by managing the psychodynamics of drug prescribing (Chapter 8); elevating the goals by bending the standard rules of therapy (Chapter 9); understanding the genesis of internal saboteurs and other dissociated subpersonalities and the means of integrating them into a unified self; and utilizing the outpatient therapeutic community to overcome borderline instability of relationships and to achieve intimacy (Chapter 11). In the final chapter, I look closely at the possibility of achieving creativity and freedom, the richest fruits of the work.

ACKNOWLEDGMENTS

I am indebted to many teachers and colleagues for the ideas and clinical experiences that inform this book. Since I have often adapted their contributions to my own purposes, however, they must be absolved of any responsibility for the final form they have taken here. With this proviso, I must express my gratitude to Elvin Semrad, Carl Whitaker, Salvador Minuchin, and Robert Pottash for making me aware of the artistic possibilities of a psychodynamically attuned existential therapy. And to Joseph Kepecs I give thanks for a rich and humane introduction to the world of the Freudian unconscious. In addition, I am grateful to Kohut's self psychology which has become so woven into the fabric of my thought that I am no longer able to give adequate acknowledgment of its influence.

A very special debt must be paid to Milton H. Miller, who was Chairman of the Department of Psychiatry at the University of Wisconsin when I taught there in the late 1960s and early 1970s. To my knowledge, Dr. Miller ran the only existential department in the annals of modern medicine, and he served as my main mentor in adopting the existential therapy perspective. He was also responsible for making me aware of the workings of internal saboteurs in human affairs and thus responsible for one of the major causal principles of the therapeutic approach developed here. Finally, more than any single individual, he demonstrated the nature of the projection of will involved in publishing one's ideas.

My colleague Richard Hole has generously given his time in reading the manuscript in its various drafts. His critiques have always been thoughtful and incisive. My cotherapist, Mary R. E. Leshan, has been of invaluable assistance in running the groups that form the core of the therapeutic milieu and in providing adjunctive individual therapy for those patients suffering from severe maternal deprivation. I am indebted to my editor, Carol Stillman, for her sensitive guidance in improving the syntax and the clarity of my thought. She has been a kind, attuned companion throughout the whole journey of putting the book together.

Finally, I must give thanks to my patients, who have endured my mistakes and repeatedly given me another chance to help them climb the steps to freedom. I am privileged to have worked with so many dedicated and forgiving human beings, who were able to take the limited help I had to offer and then to work their way to a higher plane of mental and physical health.

EUGENE M. ABROMS, M.D.

Ardmore, Pennsylvania

Contents

CHAPTER 1

The Bio-Existential Spirit

Psychotherapy is beginning to change its tune. It used to value intellectual insight and moral neutrality above all else. But with the appearance of newer techniques and sicker patients, stronger, more penetrating chords are now being struck. This is nowhere more evident than in the behavior of therapists. They once delivered their carefully measured interpretations to neurotics from behind the couch. Now they enter actively into the world of borderlines and psychotics, banging hard on their character armor and sewing up splits in the self. Not content merely to ask why, they also show how. In the process, therapy goes beyond free association to determined interaction. The spirit of this new approach is captured in an old hasidic tale, which I have recast as a modern therapy parable.[1]

After the Vietnam War, an emaciated soldier, shattered by the brutality of his experiences, returned home and slipped into psychosis. He developed delusion that he was a bird. Wearing only a blue pair of briefs, he perched on windowsills and tabletops, periodically chirping and flapping his arms. He had hallucinations of soaring in flight. He refused to touch the meats and vegetables that his mother anxiously served; instead, he would drink only water and eat only nuts and seeds. No amount of pleading would get him to behave normally.

His parents took the soldier to a psychiatrist, who made the diagnosis of psychosis and had him hospitalized. The hospital stay and the prescribed medication diminished but did not cure his symptoms: He spoke less often and seemed less certain of his delusions, but they would flare up in times of stress. When he was discharged home on medication and with reassurances that he was getting well, his parents were dissatisfied, because they wanted their son back exactly as he had been before the war. Fortunately, the discharge team made a careful referral, sending the patient to an innovative therapist, also a Vietnam veteran, who made house calls in special cases.

At the appointed time the therapist came right to the patient's home and asked to be shown to his room. Upon entering and finding him undressed on the windowsill, the therapist immediately stripped down to his underwear and joined the man on the perch.

"What the hell are you doing?" asked the patient.

"And you," replied the therapist, "what the hell are you doing?"

"Can't you see? I am a bird, and this is my perch."

"Well, I'm a bird, too, and I'm perching here with you."

Quite surprisingly, they began to hit it off. In fact, their conversation became contagious. They made plans to visit together again, and soon were doing it regularly. One day while they were exchanging old war stories, the therapist casually slipped on his shirt. The young veteran was flabbergasted.

"Have you lost touch with reality, dressing in men's clothes? Have you forgotten that you are a bird? You must have an unresolved wish to be a man."

"You're much too psychological about this. A man can dress in a gorilla suit without wanting to be a gorilla, and a bird can dress in human clothing without wishing to be or thinking he is a man. A bird in men's clothing is clearly still a bird."

After careful reflection, the patient conceded the point. The next day both dressed in their regular pants and shirts. Sometime later, the therapist ordered a humus-on-pita from the kitchen.

"Now look what you're doing! This is clearly a major regression. You're beginning to eat like them."

"And you are going overboard again. Just because you eat human food doesn't make you a human being, any more than eating Lebanese food makes you Lebanese. You can eat anything you want with anybody you choose and still remain the bird you are."

The former combat soldier, who had witnessed many atrocities and been told many lies, could not deafen himself to the right of truth. He started sleeping in his bed again and joining his family for meals. He even resumed singing and playing the piano, which he had not done in years. That fall he enrolled in college as a music major. In the spring he took the part of Papageno in a modern staging of *The Magic Flute*. He fell in love with his Papageno and began to think seriously about the future. The therapist came for the final performance and with great rejoicing rang down the curtain on the veteran's illness.

There are many points that could be made about this story, but just as in the type of therapy that it depicts, interpretations are often more effective if they are enacted rather than verbalized. Yet the most basic idea can be said quite simply and directly: that the therapist in the tale is highly interactive with the patient and joins him mentally and physically in the world of his psychosis. He closes the distance between them by first sitting on the same perch and only later leading him back to the dinner table and everyday reality. This is what is so "existential" about his approach. Moreover, beyond therapeutic tactics, he truly has a greater deal in common with the patient. They are both veterans of the same war, and this creates an intuitive understanding between them that obviates the usual need for self-explanations. Implicitly, the therapist was similarly scarred by his combat experiences and thus can strongly empathize with how the patient has also been wounded. But he has clearly healed himself, because he is now capable of rejoicing in his charge's renewed health and creativity—just as he earlier joined him in his sickness. First he makes a house call, and then later a real-life call.

Notice also that he tears nothing down, only adding to what he finds in a way that transforms it. He does not interpretively attack the patient's delusions but rather treats them as manifestations of a higher truth that needs to be properly clothed. Nor does he throw out the patient's past treatment. He neither discontinues the medication nor discounts the diagnosis of his colleagues, but instead builds on them to make his own intervention. In fact, the success of his approach depends on the prior impact of the medical approach. Because it is a combination of biomedical and existential therapy, it is truly *bio-existential,* to coin an oxymoron.

But this is a clinical parable, not a real case history. We must now see how actual patients are treated in the bio-existential mode. There are critical differences. In clinical practice, clients suffer less from ornithological delusions than from failures in their love and work lives. And therapists do not strip down to their underwear; they find more appropriate ways of getting close that do not risk overexposure. Finally, real bio-existential therapy integrates not only the biomedical and existential dimensions of treatment but the vast psychosocial ground that ties between them. In this sense, the term itself is short for bio-psycho-socio-existential.[2] The following case report is meant to explore the linkages within this long train of ideas.

Larry, a corporate recruiter in his late 30s, was referred with his wife Myrna when their 2-year-old marriage, his second, began to unravel. They found themselves constantly bickering and unable to reconcile their differences. Although very sexually attracted to Myrna, who was physically beautiful, Larry was abruptly turned off soon after their marriage when she complained at great length about the paltriness of the wedding presents and the stinginess of the friends and relatives who gave them. By origin a churchgoing, hardworking Midwest farm boy, Larry found the spiteful, petty materialism of Myrna's complaining highly offensive. But why had he not noticed this aspect of her character before? In truth, what exactly—surely not just the specific complaints—was driving such a sharp stake into the heart of their romance?

The most obvious factor that emerged from our couples sessions was that Myrna and Larry had very little in common besides sexual attraction. As already noted, their values were discordant, concerning not just materialism but the importance of loyalty and propriety in relationships. And their temperaments clashed: He was serious and compulsive, she brash and impulsive. Yet they lacked the mutual respect that turns the attraction of opposites into real complementarity. Although they did similar work and liked to eat out and see movies together, they had no shared spiritual commitments, such as joint involvement in a serious belief, art, or social cause. They also came from very different ethnic and religious backgrounds, and they had no common network of friends. In truth, the match between them was so poorly supported that very strong irrational forces must have operated to bring them together in the first place.

What I learned about these forces came from several joint sessions and then therapy with Larry alone while Myrna pursued her own individual treatment with a colleague; thus, my understanding is heavily weighted on Larry's side. Yet it became abundantly clear that Myrna was having severe mood swings, that she alternated between a hypersexual, intrusive overactivity (which could easily turn into abusive blaming) and inconsolate, weepy self-pity—especially when Larry became enraged at her, which he did frequently. Her psychiatrist started her on lithium coupled with psychotherapy, but this treatment, although beneficial, did not stem the tide of the marital breakup.

Why Larry, an otherwise thoughtful and responsible person, was attracted to someone with wild mood swings soon became apparent from the review of his family history. His father appeared to be manic-depressive and psychotic to boot: He oscillated between periods of hateful, morose spitefulness and grandiose outbursts of tyranny, during which he would hit Larry with shovels and stick him with pitchforks for imagined shortcomings in his farm chores. These attacks stopped only when Larry became both fast and bold enough to outrun his father. Despite this harsh mistreatment, Larry worked on the farm uncomplainingly (often from dawn to dusk) for the welfare of the family, in which he passionately believed. His depressed mother, who was loving toward him, nevertheless made excuses for her husband's behavior and masochistically absorbed the latter's abuse, leaving him only after he drew a gun on Larry's younger brother.

My understanding was that Larry, in marrying and subsequently battling with Myrna, was reliving in milder form his early family relationships, which involved being caught between a violent, cyclothymic father and a depressed, mistreated mother who were always fighting. Because both Myrna and Larry often shifted roles in this reenactment, they not only replayed Larry's relationships with each parent but the parents' sadomasochistic relationship with each other. Myrna's personality contained the required attributes to reenact these old dramas under Larry's direction.

The limitations of insight as a corrective factor, however, soon became apparent. It is one thing to recognize that one is the victim of early conditioning and quite another to stop the conditioned behavior. Once he saw how futile it was to cease fighting with Myrna while they lived together, Larry was very decisive in moving for a separation. But he conspired to keep the battle raging by continuing to get together with her, answering her many phone calls, and allowing her to come over for unannounced visits. On each occasion, an argument ensued. Finally and with reluctance, Larry became convinced that the marriage was beyond saving, and with my support he began the painful process of disconnecting. Only as he succeeded in erecting a solid barrier between himself and Myrna—for example, by never answering phones or doorbells before identifying the caller—did he begin to mourn the loss of the marriage.

In this process of disconnecting from Myrna, Larry allowed me to guide many of his actions. I advised him to buy an answering machine to monitor his phone calls. I told him "up front" that I thought he and Myrna had little in common, particularly in the realm of values. Later on, I referred him to a good accountant and financial adviser to help him manage his affairs. Why did he give me this degree of influence when, by all rights, he should have had a negative father transference? I will go further into this matter of trust later, but what was clear from the beginning was that he connected strongly with me. We both came from isolated rural farm backgrounds, we had many interests and values in common, and there was a kinship of spirit right from the start.

With my support and guidance, then, Larry disconnected from Myrna and later started the equally painful process of trying to fill the resulting void by exploring new relationships. What soon became obvious from his efforts was that he was preferentially attracted to sadistic or masochistic women. Repeatedly and uncannily Larry found himself with dates who (like his father) were either openly abusive toward him or who (like his mother) elicited his outraged, impotent sympathies with their tales of abuse by others. Try as he might to avoid such people, he could not stay away from them.

Slowly Larry began to catch himself earlier and earlier in the game, but at the same time he became aware that he was not ordinarily attracted to healthy women. They seemed bovinely dull to him! With this appalling insight, he stopped going out altogether, declaring a moratorium on dating that was to last a whole year. In an effort to buffer the loneliness of this time he joined one of my therapy groups and received the social support necessary to making major life changes. As in all successful "latency" periods, great emphasis was placed on his work. During this year, Larry left his job, where he had been (not surprisingly) treated poorly. He made the enormous investment of resources to start his own recruiting firm, out of the reach of abusive authority figures.

At the end of this phase he became involved with a worthwhile person who stood outside his neurotic pattern, who neither gave nor wanted abuse. The growing closeness with her, though, soon became intolerable. He was constantly irritated by her minor violations of his privacy, which stirred up old feelings of being violated by his father. As he, with therapeutic pressure and support, forced himself not to run away from her, however, he became clinically depressed and had to be started on antidepressant medication. The curbing of his tendency to run exposed an underlying depression and gave the first clues of the existence of an internal saboteur,[3] a part of his personality that worked against the conscious aim of achieving intimacy.

As this relationship finally succumbed to his saboteur, Larry realized that his first marriage had failed for quite similar reasons: that his wife, too, had been relatively healthy, but a part of him was intolerant of her emotional availability and therefore arranged his work schedule so that he was out of town most weekends! If he stayed at home, he found himself becoming either angry or depressed, for reasons he could not understand. When he continued this travel pattern despite her vociferous complaints, his wife finally gave up on the relationship and moved for a divorce.

Larry was now armed with the awareness that to the extent he relived the past by selecting a parental surrogate, his love life degenerated into a battle, and to the extent that his selection process was healthier, the resulting intimacy brought out a part of him that sabotaged the relationship either through distancing or by expressing rage and depression. The rage and depression, apart from their biological determinants, drew their intensity from the crucial formative event of his past history: the betrayal of his innocent love by his father's psychotic cruelty. It was this traumatic experience that caused an angry, depressed, and destructive part of the personality, an internal saboteur, to split off from the central self.

Clearly, anyone hoping to get close to Larry would be subjected to an ordeal, and therefore the attempt was only for the stouthearted. A viable candidate for his affections would have to possess a large arsenal of courage, insight, and appreciation of his decency against great odds. Fortuitously, he was introduced to Linda, who possessed these traits in abundance, just as he became ready to contend for love on a higher plane.

Linda was a hardworking therapy patient herself, having gone into treatment with a psychologist after the breakup of her marriage. Thus, she shared Larry's values as to the importance of psychological growth and owning one's part in interpersonal conflicts. As squabbles inevitably arose between them, they jointly undertook the steps that were necessary to resolve their difficulties, which included sharing their feelings very openly, having couples therapy sessions with me or Linda's therapist, and even separating for periods of time. The biggest challenge to the relationship, however, was the ever more virulent appearances of Larry's internal saboteur. Larry committed a number of acts whose main purpose seemed to be the destruction of Linda's love and respect, always at times when they had just become more intimate. He became irritable, withdrew sexually, told her about other women in his past life, or found himself too busy to see her. Worst of all, he precipitated a series of business crises that aroused fears of impending bankruptcy, casting doubts on his ability to hold up his financial end of the relationship.

True to his track record, however, Larry showed unflinching honesty and hard work in corralling his saboteur. With Linda's cooperation and the help of individual, couples, and group therapy, he caught himself earlier and earlier in the act of acting out. He grabbed his saboteur by the throat, as it were, and gradually induced it to work for him instead of against him—a topic I will explore more fully in Chapter 10. In the process, he looked at his fear of surpassing his brutal father and becoming fully and independently successful; he gained real understanding of the identification and dissociation processes that led to the formation of his split-off saboteur; and he came to see why this part of himself was so hurt and destructively angry and what was involved in assuaging its feelings.

In her therapy, Linda worked hard on diminishing her contribution to arguments and conflicts with Larry. When his business appeared to be going under and he could no longer afford help, she offered to answer the phones and do data entry for him on a temporary basis. Gradually she got involved with clients and soon asked Larry to train her as his office manager, for which she showed great aptitude. Despite an intensification of their arguments, Linda's coming to work improved Larry's sense of optimism and comfort at the office. Business began to improve, and he was soon out of financial danger. He drew special meaning from the fact that it was now a common venture, just as the family farm on which he had worked diligently for the first 18 years of his life was supposed to have been. Moreover, he was deeply moved by Linda's drive to excel in both her personal and professional development. With his help, she made the moves toward health and competence that he had always coveted for his mother and father.

Yet, as he was on the brink of getting everything he wanted, the remaining vestiges of the cruel father inside him made one last vicious attempt to destroy his world. Going for the jugular of his love alliance, his dangerously weakened saboteur started lashing out at Linda's mistakes on the job, reaching such a peak of petty meanness as to either crush her spirit or drive her away. Completely excoriating the remnants of this persistent demon involved corrective feedback and support from his group and myself and his own willingness to look at and neutralize his hateful part. Rather than attacking him for its nastiness, I acknowledged his past accomplishments in therapy and reaffirmed my faith in his ability to surmount his hurdle as well. Thus, I provided a model of how he should respond to Linda's mistakes, on terms that were vastly different from his father's abuse. Once this storm subsided, Larry and Linda made plans to move in together and explore the possibility of a more lasting, intimate relationship.

What we see in this case are the multitude of factors that impaired Larry's ability to live intimately and, therefore, the many types of repairs that had to be made. First of all, he doomed his love life from the very start by picking unsuitable partners. The legacy of his brutal upbringing was that he often chose either sadistic or masochistic women and then reenacted abusive relationships with them. But the healthy part of his personality rebelled against this outcome. Thus, psychotherapy had to start by getting him, through insight and retraining, to stop getting involved with the "wrong" people. But once he accomplished this, a new, even higher hurdle had to be scaled: developing an attraction for suitable partners, who were at first unappealing to him. This involved a painful moratorium on all dating, followed by a gradual exposure to new kinds of activities and people. Once this process pushed Larry toward more appropriate matches, an obviously destructive part of his personality came out, one that seemed intent on destroying all possibility of successful love and work in his life. Neutralizing this internal saboteur and getting it to become an ally instead of an enemy thus became the final stage of his treatment.

Both psychodynamic insight and cognitive and behavioral relearning were necessary components of the broad-gauged psychotherapy that taught Larry how to love effectively. But they were not the only responsible factors. Patients who confront and curb the acting out of their internal saboteurs almost always become clinically depressed. As the reader will see in subsequent chapters, the whole purpose of splitting off a part of the personality is to diminish an intolerable feeling of grief. Therefore, reining in the saboteur (by blocking off its channels of acting out) reevokes the original state of overwhelming depression. To get through this experience, antidepressants and other mood stabilizers may have to be prescribed, as they were in Larry's case. Only in this way can the original grief be diminished enough to be faced.

But medicines are not enough. There is also a need for a wide web of emotional support, and this is where the social therapies come in. Larry benefited from both couples and group therapy in getting his love and work lives straightened out. He received encouragement and feedback from myself, Linda, and his fellow group members. It is doubtful that this man, who grew up on an isolated farm with no close friends, could have faced the pain of extensive personality change without an extensive support group, which he was unable to generate on his own. Moreover, as the reader will see in Chapter 4, group therapy can be further organized to provide an outpatient therapeutic community that can work effectively to stabilize the relationships of patients who cannot otherwise form lasting bonds.

Finally, internal saboteurs cannot simply be extinguished or conditioned away. They have to be replaced. The part of a saboteur that represents a bad introject, such as Larry's identification with his psychotically cruel father, has to be supplanted by an appropriate role model. Serving as such a model—as the good ego ideal that drives out the bad introject—involves the therapist in becoming the patient's mentor. Rather than being a technician who provides only intellectual insights or behavioral prescriptions, the therapist as mentor must also serve as practical helper and moral guide, showing the patient the ropes of life. It is often with a painful sense of inadequacy that we therapists try to fill this existential role. For all our limitations, patients tend to accept us as "good enough" guides if we approach the task with appropriate competence and humility.

In Larry's case, I served as a parental model by directly offering support and guidance for many of his life changes. For him to accept my influence, however, he had to come to trust me. This he did for several important reasons. First of all, my advice and example proved reasonably reliable and helpful. I had already been through many of the same life changes that Larry was experiencing, and coming from a similar hardworking rural background, I had an immediate understanding of and sympathy for his worldview. Second, I made it clear that even though I was glad to give advice, he was under no obligation to take it; in fact, I preferred that he come up with his own solutions, which I would defer to and support to the best of my ability. As he became stronger, I increasingly adopted the nondirective stance of the traditional therapist. These are crucial adjustments for any activist therapy that also seeks to foster the patient's autonomy and independence. Third, I liked and respected him greatly, and I made no secret of it. I thought he had risen above great adversity to become a very decent human being. I looked up to him for his decency and integrity.

For these and other reasons Larry came to trust me, even allowing me initially to guide his relationship with Linda, which (given his past history of broken love affairs) had little chance of surviving without special outside help. He learned to love her in a stable way, bolstered by many deeply shared values and a common business venture. To accomplish this goal, Larry underwent the whole gamut of existing psychiatric treatments: group, individual psychodynamic, cognitive and behavior, marital and family, and psychoactive drug therapies. Moreover, great attention was paid to the existential aspects of psychotherapy: the necessity for therapist and patient, and patient and loved ones, to develop common values, to share a strong belief system whose ideals serve as self-fulfilling prophecies of mutual growth.

What I want to do in the pages ahead is to provide a rationale for integrating all the major approaches to therapy, as I have done in Larry's case, and to give further examples of how the resulting pluralistic and activist treatment makes it possible for patients with severe personality disorders to develop stable intimacy. This mode of therapy is not the recommended approach for ordinary neurotic disorders, which can usually be managed by less intrusive methods. But for high functioning borderline patients, whose ability to earn an adequate living is not accompanied by comparable success in sustaining close ties, it may offer the best chance for leading a meaningful life.

NOTES

1. This fable derives from Rabbi Nachman of Bratzlav's tale of the prince and the rooster. See Elie Wiesel's traditional version, to which I am indebted, in *Souls on Fire* (New York: Random House, 1972, pp. 170-171). The film *Birdy* (Columbia Pictures, 1985) also influenced me in modernizing the tale.
2. This boxcarlike term derives from *biopsychosocial,* the adjective coined by George Engel to denote the posteclectic, pluralistic paradigm that modern medicine and psychiatry are moving toward. See G. L. Engel, "The Need for a New Medical Model: A Challenge for Biomedicine," *Science 196:*129–136, 1977.
3. The notion of an internal saboteur has obvious roots in ancient ideas of demon possession. Its modern formulation, as the reader will see in the next chapter, derives from 19th-century French conceptions of personality dissociation. I first encountered the term *internal saboteur* in the context of Ronald Fairbairn's object relations theory. See W. R. D. Fairbairn, *Psychoanalytic Studies of the Personality,* London: Routledge and Kegan Paul, 1952, pp. 82–161.

CHAPTER 2

The Definition and History of Psychotherapy

The history of psychotherapy covers a vast canvas, stretching back to prehistoric man's first rituals for propitiating the gods and then forward to the medieval worshiper's ceremonies for exorcising his demons. Toward its cutting edge one can observe a multigenerational family meeting in which the kinship tries to exorcise demons of a very modern sort: failures in love leading to hurts and injustices that are passed down through the generations of the family's life. Psychotherapy has a rich history, one that is often overwhelming in its abundant testimonies to man's complexity. The symptomatic manifestations of failed love are so varied as to appear ornate in their invention. But they are no less so than the methods concocted for their relief, which range from whirling dervishes to whirling chairs, from mortification of the flesh to quiet contemplation. Because of its myriad forms, the attempt to provide psychotherapy with a unifying definition cannot entirely succeed, but good work has nevertheless been done in coming up with one. We must review this effort and see what amendments are needed.

DEFINITION OF PSYCHOTHERAPY

Jerome Frank made the major breakthrough in defining psychotherapy in his classic work, *Persuasion and Healing*.[1] According to him, psychotherapy is a structural series of contacts between a socially sanctioned healer and a mental sufferer. Through these contacts the healer, often with the aid of a group, tries to produce positive changes in the sufferer's emotional state, attitudes, and behavior. Although physical and chemical adjuncts may be used, the healing influence is primarily exercised by words, acts, and rituals.[2]

The major elements of his definition—the structured contacts, the socially sanctioned healer, and the influence of words, acts, and rituals—will occupy us throughout this book. The structured nature of psychotherapy finds expression in its many rules, such as having a fixed duration and frequency of sessions. The purpose and flexible utilization of these rules will be a major topic of the discussion in Chapter 9. The social prestige of the healer and his or her reliance on words, acts, and rituals are so germane to the history of psychotherapy that one must address their significance right away. These characteristics establish a connection between psychotherapy and other types of psychic influence, particularly religious and magical healing.

This connection is one of the major theses of Frank's work. He shows how psychotherapy, faith healing, religious conversion ceremonies, placebo administration, and even brainwashing techniques are all influencing operations, methods of persuading people to change their values and their outlook on themselves and the world. In so doing, they overcome anxiety, depression, and even symptoms of physical illness—the bitterest fruits of failed love—and they do so by replacing them with positive beliefs that generate hope and meaning.

For such persuasion to occur, the healer must have personal magnetism or social prestige, preferably both. In addition, he must (through words, acts, and rituals) utilize this power to inspire faith in the sufferer that some suprapersonal force or process can be made to act on his behalf. In other words, the healer must be able to engender positive expectations of benefit by instilling faith in a belief system that promises rewards in return for observance. This process is helped immeasurably by the presence of a group of believers who exert social pressure to join their ranks and who provide living examples of the healing power of believing and belonging. This confession of past sins and sufferings and the acceptance of the sinner by the healer and the group despite his or her past behavior are also potent facilitators of this healing by faith.

Fortified by this framework, we can look at both religious healing and psychotherapy with fresh eyes. We can understand better the rituals and ceremonial gatherings presided over by shamans, witch doctors, and medicine men[3] and why these have proven helpful to primitive people. The role of etiological explanations, such as loss of soul or intrusion of foreign spirits, even when they are patently false, falls into place as a factor in promoting relief from suffering. In the modern religions of the Western world, we can appreciate better the healing properties of common worship, confession of sins, appeals to divine intervention, indoctrination, and symbolic rituals.[4]

Modern psychotherapy also has its prestigious healers, its belief systems appealing to suprapersonal forces, its methods of indoctrination, and its healing rituals. Psychotherapy, no less than faith healing and brainwashing, is a method of persuasion leading to relief of mental suffering. And quite clearly, psychotherapy not only has much in common with religious healing but is its major historical descendant. Apart from their common procedures, the ideas of leading theorists of psychotherapy (particularly Freud and Jung) have been increasingly scrutinized in recent times for their debt, largely unacknowledged, to the mystical traditions of the great religions.[5]

Psychotherapy, then, is a method of persuasion. But is that all it is? Although Frank does not address this question in any detail, it is clearly an important issue, because the legitimacy of the undertaking hinges on it. Neither as therapists nor as patients would we be content to make the huge investments required for psychotherapy were it no more than a method of faith healing, indoctrination, or placebo administration. The evidence that it is more has accumulated quite massively over the past half century. The charge that it is only an inert placebo has been most decisively laid to rest; there are now close to 500 controlled studies demonstrating the efficacy of psychotherapy.[6] The methodological rigor of this validation process meets the highest standards of scientific truth in the behavioral sciences.

The charge that psychotherapy is no more than healing by faith can also be convincingly answered. What one must develop faith in to be healed by psychotherapy is that bad habits learned in the past can be unlearned, conflicts that have impeded psychological development can be resolved, and that some maladaptive behaviors have out-of-awareness determinants that can be modified. Contrary to ordinary faith healing, no appeal to supernatural causes is made. In fact, the majority of the explanations invoked are empirically verifiable, at least in principle. The faith required for modern psychotherapy, therefore, is a faith in modern naturalistic science, and healing by that kind of faith is more than acceptable; it is the only rational belief. Any claims of healing by other means should be regarded with great skepticism.

Similarly, the notion that psychotherapy is an indoctrination procedure analogous to brainwashing can also be countered. An indoctrination voluntarily sought out and voluntarily continued may be persuasive but hardly coercive, and the difference is a major one. Brainwashing is, by definition, coercive. Psychotherapy in the modern sense ceases to exist when its patients are forced to continue it, when they are not free to come and go. Its spirit is violated when, short of coercion, intense social pressure is exerted on its behalf and banishment is threatened for doctrinal dissent. Finally, the assent that is sought is not to any ordinary ideology but to hypotheses susceptible to empirical testing. This kind of indoctrination is what we commonly mean by education. With respect to formal learning, there is no acceptable alternative.

So we can grant that psychotherapy has elements in common with faith healing, indoctrination, and placebo response, but also that it goes beyond these other methods of persuasion to base its validity on the acquisition of objective knowledge by voluntary means. In saying this, however, we have not quite gotten to the heart of the matter. There is an issue about psychotherapy that I have skirted, that those of us who want to retain the mantle of scientific respectability always tend to skirt. It is the matter of out-of-awareness motivation. The workings of the unconscious mind have not been emphasized in this discussion, nor in Frank's, because its effects and therapeutic management, inherently subjective, are so difficult to discuss and document by objective means. We are on less solid scientific ground here, as evidenced by the level of controversy among serious students of the field as to the role of unconscious factors in symptom formation and treatment.

Yet it is quite clear from the history of psychotherapy that its modern development coincides with the naturalistic exploration of unconscious mental processes. In fact, the theory of modern psychotherapy begins when healers stop attributing mental causation to supernatural agencies and instead locate it exclusively in the intrapersonal and interpersonal spheres. And the practice of modern psychotherapy starts when therapists realize that what had been regarded as supernatural actually comes, at least in part, from the natural part of the self that is unconscious. Then therapists could learn to influence these unconscious processes directly without appealing to supernatural mediation. A selective review of this history provides a useful perspective from which to regard the approach to psychotherapy outlined in this book. In the discussion that follows I am most indebted to Ellenberger's monumental study, *The Discovery of the Unconscious.*[7] The works of Zilboorg[8] and Mora[9] have also proven helpful.

THE MODERN HISTORY

By general agreement, the history of modern psychiatry begins in the sixteenth century with the contributions of Paracelsus (c. 1493–1541) and Johann Weyer (1515–1588). These two eminent physicians started the whole process of medicalizing mental illness and its treatment, a process still in progress. The Swiss doctor Paracelsus pointed out that there are diseases of the body and diseases "which deprive man of his reason," and that these latter are not, as the clergy claim, attributable to "ghostly beings and three-fold spirits." Rather, "nature is the sole origin of diseases," and the mental patient is neither a criminal nor a sinner, but a sick person in need of medical treatment.[10] Similarly, Weyer undercut the witch-hunting craze fostered by Sprenger and Kramer's infamous diatribe of 1486, *Malleus Maleficarum*,[11] by vehemently rejecting the belief in witchcraft and chastising the clergy for supporting it. He showed how the presumed signs and symptoms of witchcraft were, in the main, explainable in medical terms.[12] Both Weyer and Paracelsus advocated the practice of psychotherapy for such victims of mental illness, a psychotherapy based mainly on benevolent understanding and counseling. Quite remarkably, both also invoked the operation of unconscious motivation in producing symptoms. In the case of Barbara Kremers, who claimed to subsist for over a year without food or drink, Weyer moved the patient into his own home for observation and treatment. He discovered that she was sneaking food during the night but could not acknowledge it. He concluded that the patient's behavior represented an "unconscious desire to malinger." Similarly, Paracelsus attributed the cause of St. Vitus's dance or "chorea lascivà" to unconscious ideas, in what Zilboorg claims to be the first mention of unconscious motivation of neurosis in the history of medical psychology.[13]

Mesmer and the Mesmerists

The first explicitly medical technique (i.e., one invoking natural versus supernatural or religious means) for treating neurosis was discovered by Franz Anton Mesmer (1734–1815) on July 28, 1774.[14] At this time, while treating Fraulein Oesterlin for multiple, debilitating somatic complaints, Mesmer—inspired by some English physicians' experiments with magnets—sought to create an "artificial tide" by having the patient swallow iron filings and attaching magnets to various parts of her body. The patient began to experience a stream of mysterious fluid running through her body, which swept away all her symptoms for several hours and subsequently led to a complete recovery (eventuating in marriage to Mesmer's stepson and raising a family). Mesmer located the healing influence not in the magnets alone but in the mysterious bodily fluid, whose effects the external magnets only directed. He called this healing tide "animal magnetism," and he spent the rest of his tumultuous life trying to explain its workings and developing the words, acts, and rituals to maximize its effective utilization. The very next year (1775), Mesmer engaged in his celebrated "treatment duel" with Gassner, the most renowned exorcist of the day, in which Mesmer demonstrated that Gassner's cures could all be achieved by animal magnetism without reference to God or the devil. The obvious implication of Mesmer's victory was that Gassner, no matter how he himself accounted for his healing effects, was in fact relying on animal magnetism.

It fell to one of Mesmer's greatest followers, the Marquis de Puységur (1751–1825), to correct Mesmer's mistake as to the nature of personal magnetism. Puységur, member of a noble family of French military commanders and amateur scientists, established that magnetic influence occurred most effectively in an altered state of consciousness that he termed "artificial somnambulism," now known as hypnotic trance. In the trance state, the subject appears both asleep and hyperaware, capable of self-diagnosis and projecting the future but amnesic about the trance when later awakened. Magnetism, according to Puységur, is exerted not through any fluid but entirely psychologically (i.e., by virtue of the will and beliefs of the participants).[15]

Four other main features of the trance state, although known to Puységur and Mesmer, were worked out more fully by their continental protégés.[16] The first is that magnetic influence is best exerted in a state of *rapport* between magnetist and subject, a state of heightened psychological attunement. It is this mutual empathy that facilitates the induction of the trance state and the subject's willingness to respond to the directives given in it. As the reader will see, the subsequent history of psychotherapy can be regarded as an elaboration of this point, a moving away from trying to influence solely by intimidation toward doing it by affectionate concern. From this perspective, modern psychotherapy represents a movement away from an impositional hypnotherapy toward a collaborative one.

The second discovery of the mesmerists about the trance state is that directives given during trance are typically carried out in the waking state without memory of the origins of the behavior—without awareness, to put it boldly, that one is still partially in trance and only apparently fully awake. As will be discussed shortly, this awareness of the phenomena of posthypnotic suggestion paved the way for Charcot's work on the production of experimental neuroses and Janet, Breuer, and Freud's elucidation of the role of the psychocatharsis of unconscious experiences in resolving neurotic symptoms. A forgotten memory of an experience could produce current symptoms, according to these pioneers, and its recovery from its buried sleep-state could rid the patient of his or her symptoms.

Related to this point is the third finding: Puységur's great intuition that mental illness is itself a negative trance state, negative in the sense that a part of the personality is "asleep" and inaccessible to the self, which is consequently diminished in its richness and potency. Obviously, then, the cure of neurosis and psychosis involves an awakening from a constricted trance state by the induction of a deconstricting, positive trance. Our current notion that some neurotic symptoms are dissociated, entranced parts of the self is foreshadowed in this idea, as is the obvious treatment strategy suggested by it—the induction of an altered state aimed at the integration of the self.

The fourth observation of the mesmerists about the somnambulist state is that while in it, subjects tend to manifest multiple personalities.[17] In other words, their bodies appear to become inhabited by other "persons" with names and characters entirely different from the normal, waking self. The realization that these multiple personalities are all dissociated parts of the one self and not inhabitations by other selves culminated in Freud's division of the personality into the subpersonalities of ego, id, and superego and Jung's subdivision of it into such archetypes as the *anima* and *animus*. It should be noted that Freud's three structures do not have enough "personality," as he described them, to explain how an individual can have an internal saboteur or protector, a harmful or helpful agent that is capable of influencing total psychosomatic behavior. It was left to Fairbairn and other English theorists to elucidate the role of these part-subjects.

The French School

Jean-Martin Charcot (1825–1893), the foremost neurologist of the nineteenth century, studied the phenomena of hysteria and hypnosis experimentally and thereby conferred academic respectability on these subjects.[18] With him, neurosis moved to the center stage of psychiatry, and with neurosis on the stage, the unconscious became the main player. Charcot demonstrated that an unconscious idea could be the cause of a neurotic symptom: a hysterical paralysis, seizure, pain, anesthesia, or amnesia. Using hypnosis he suggested such symptoms, which could then be made to appear and disappear at his command during the waking state (in the absence of the gross organic lesions responsible for such symptoms on a traumatic or degenerative basis). Charcot also established the close connection between hysteria and hypnosis, but in the process he overstated the case. He thought that only hysterics could be hypnotized, thereby allocating all hypnotic phenomena to the realm of the pathological. Charcot missed out on the possibility that hypnosis had etiological and treatment implications for all neurotics, not just hysterics.

Because of his recognition of this fact, Hippolyte Bernheim (1840–1919), who with his mentor Liébeault founded the Nancy school of psychiatry, is credited by Zilboorg with being Freud's immediate precursor as the founder of modern dynamic psychotherapy.[19] Bernheim discovered that nonhysterical neurotics and normals could be hypnotized and relieved of psychosomatic symptoms by hypnotic suggestion. Even more importantly, he discovered that these hypnotic psychotherapeutic effects could be achieved in the waking state, without putting the patient in trance. In one sense, Freud's achievement as the originator of a modern psychotherapy is an elaboration of this discovery by Bernheim: What is the psychoanalytic method if not a subtle, effective form of hypnotic suggestion in the guise of a thoroughly rational therapy? Where Charcot did prove more of a precursor to Freud and the other depth psychologists than Bernheim, however, was in the former's recognition that the study of artistic creations, no less than the study of the mentally ill, could provide invaluable insights into psychopathology, as evidenced by his studies of artistic expression with Richer.[20]

Pierre Janet (1859–1947) is considered by modern students of psychotherapy to be the most underrated pioneer of the psychodynamic approach.[21] The reasons are not mysterious; unlike Freud, he was no poet, and therefore he provides much less fascination for the reader. Moreover, he did not inspire a zealous band of followers to stake out exclusive claims to his intellectual territory. And for reasons of personality, he did not passionately own and proclaim the revolutionary import of his ideas. Perhaps these are all reflections of the fact that his theory has a certain static quality; it does not dip into the wellspring of human motives, the very heart of Freud's work.

Nevertheless, Janet's contributions were major. He propounded the doctrine of subconscious fixed ideas as the source of neurotic symptoms, and he demonstrated a method for discovering these ideas (by automatic writing or automatic talking) that strikingly anticipated Freud's technique of free association. A few years before Breuer and Freud, he discovered the cathartic method of resolving these subconscious fixed ideas as the means of curing neurotic and even some psychotic symptoms. He accomplished these feats with the aid of hypnotic suggestion in both the trance and waking states.

Janet divided neurosis into "hysteria" and "psychasthenia."[22] He attributed the symptoms of hysteria to an interplay of biological and psychogenic factors. The biological predisposition resulted in "narrowing the field of consciousness," the tendency to dissociate and repress under stress. The psychogenic influence was exerted by the specific subconscious fixed ideas (what were later to become the Jungian complexes) that formed during the narrowing of consciousness.

In discussing psychasthenia, his term for depressive-obsessive neurosis, Janet introduced the notion of level of psychological tension and maintained that a whole range of neurotic symptoms resulted from a *lowering* of it, that is, from a depression of psychic energy. It is also clear that Janet regarded this lowering of the mental level as the common element responsible for all psychiatric symptoms, including hysterical and psychasthenic neurosis and even psychosis. The prominence he gives to raising the psychic energy level is consistent with the importance he ascribes to this etiological theory. This view places Janet as an early proponent of the theory I shall propose in Chapter 7: that ego-deficit grief and depression, more crucially than the ego-conflict anxiety of Freudian theory, is the virtually universal substrate of mental symptoms, and overcoming depression is often the first step in instituting any psychiatric treatment.

The Unconscious: High and Low

Before we can proceed to a full appreciation of what Freud and his dissident followers added to the history of psychotherapy, we must pick up the central theme of modern psychotherapy ushered in by Mesmer: discovering the unconscious mind and learning to influence it by hypnotic suggestion. One of Janet's early, great contributions was to review the history of hypnosis up to the end of the nineteenth century and to rediscover how much his mesmerist forebears had learned about the subconscious. By the turn of the century, the unconscious had become a widespread and lively topic of discussion, initially because of its serious treatment in the philosophies of Leibniz, Schopenhauer, Nietzsche, and von Hartmann. In experimental psychology, Fechner studied unconscious perception, Helmholtz discovered unconscious interpretation and the formation of perceptual gestalts, and Chevreuil demonstrated the influence of unconscious wishes on fine motor movements.[23]

In England in 1882, the Society for Psychical Research was founded, and one of its leaders, Frederick Myers, made a systematic study of the "subliminal self" (as he called the unconscious) in an effort to understand parapsychological phenomena.[24] Myers maintained that the subliminal self has both inferior and superior functions. The inferior ones were studied by psychopathologists in connection with the processes of dissociation and repression, what Janet called the narrowing of consciousness and the formation of subconscious fixed ideas. This was the part of the unconscious that Freud later mapped out. The superior part, according to Myers, was revealed in works of artistic and scientific genius, which represented a "subliminal uprush" of reservoirs of memories, feelings, pictures, and conceptions. As Myers also discussed, related to this function is the "mythopoetic" property of the higher unconscious: the tendency to weave fantasies, tell stories, and write poems.

Freud attempted to reduce this creative, higher part of the unconscious to nothing more than sublimations of the lower part, while Jung was to follow Myers in giving the creative unconscious an independent status. Myers also felt that the higher unconscious could occasionally get in touch with the souls of the deceased, an idea with connections to the Romantic notion that our individual souls can make contact with the world soul. This line of thought led to much discussion among nineteenth-century philosophers and hypnotists as to whether the individual unconscious was an open or a closed system, that is, whether it had access to the contents of other minds or whether its contents derived solely from the individual mind's experiences. By and large, Freud was a closed system theorist, and Jung an open system one.[25]

In 1889, Héricourt published his important survey of the unconscious contents and functions of the mind.[26] He pointed out that the conscious and unconscious minds can coexist in three states: peaceful collaboration, in which the unconscious is a silent partner; estrangement, in which the unconscious may organize into a second personality or multiple personalities, which may reveal themselves during hypnosis or in times of stress; and open rebellion, during which the struggle for control (the conflict between the conscious and unconscious) may be manifested in phobias, obsessions, compulsions, and other neurotic symptoms, eventuating in psychosis if the unconscious succeeds in completely overthrowing the governance of the conscious mind. Like all useful classifications, this one organizes a tremendous wealth of clinical material, and allows the clinician to see more clearly the therapeutic task—to overcome the estrangement or rebellion of the unconscious and to promote a fully collaborative organization of the personality.

Theodore Flournoy (1854–1920), a psychiatrist working in Geneva at the very time that Janet, Breuer, and Freud were making their discoveries of abreactive catharsis, made a lasting contribution to understanding unconscious processes by an exhaustive study of psychic mediums.[27] Flournoy demonstrated that the mediums' purported examples of clairvoyance, speaking in ancient tongues, and prior incarnations represented the unconscious reworking of forgotten early memories, often derived from books read and conversations heard. The "guiding spirits" who the mediums regarded as external good fairies were no more than their own dissociated, constructive subpersonalities.

In addition to the ability to weave "subliminal romances" (related to Myers's mythopoetic function), Flournoy attributed to the unconscious other creative abilities, such as making scientific discoveries. For example, Kekulé's dream of a snake swallowing its own tail was the inspiration behind his elucidation of the chemical structure of the benzene ring and the establishment of organic chemistry as a viable field. In its other creative functions, the unconscious can give protective warnings of danger, comfort after losses, methods for repairing blunders, and consoling, playful imaginings.

In contrast to Freud, Flournoy's emphasis here, like Myers's, is clearly on the higher, creative unconscious. Although Freudians would call for an application of Occam's razor to such expansive theorizing, modern exponents of a higher unconscious, like Jung and Assagioli,[28] would point to the reductive nature of the Freudian conception. But what neither Myers nor Flournoy fully appreciated about the unconscious, and what Freud in one of his greatest insights pointed out, is that the unconscious is essentially dynamic—it strives to get its way and therefore resists being made conscious of its own thrust, because such awareness could curb its spontaneous expression. The unconscious is thus willful in Schopenhauer's sense: a blind, brute force that wants to stay that way.[29] This is an idea that Otto Rank was to develop brilliantly, as the reader will see shortly.

What becomes clear from this survey is that prior to Freud's revolutionary discoveries, many of the elements of modern dynamic psychotherapy had already been pieced together. These included an appreciation of the role of unconscious processes, particularly as organized into multiple superpersonalities, in determining human behavior; a reasonably detailed inventory of the unconscious repertoire and the consequent redundancy of supernatural explanations; the uses of hypnosis and suggestive influence in removing unconscious pathogenic ideas and reintegrating split-off subpersonalities; the importance of the rapport between healer and sufferer in effecting therapeutic change; and the possibility of exerting the healing influence in the waking state, that is, without putting the patient in a trance.

Freud's Theory

What, then, did Freud add to these assembled ingredients? To state the answer in baldest terms, he added a powerful theory. It is a theory of unusual comprehensiveness and parsimony, comparable to Kant's critical idealism and Hegel's historicism in its explanatory power. It also shares with these other systems of thought a remarkable capacity to explain away rival theories. To criticize Freudian interpretations is, at the least, to appear defensive and, quite often, to open oneself up to being influenced by them. Freud's ideas and metaphors are so powerful that one must ignore them completely to avoid taking their suggestions. In fact, psychoanalytic theory has given birth to a belief system and a mythology that for most intellectuals of the twentieth century have performed the same function as those provided by religion in the past: providing the ethical and metaphysical underpinnings for the human enterprise.

The theory has made such a great claim on the modern imagination because it accomplishes a necessary act of synthesis, namely, the incorporation of Darwin's discoveries about evolution into the fields of psychology and psychopathology.[30] It adopts the developmental viewpoint in explaining mental symptoms. This viewpoint was already present, in primitive form, in the psychiatric writings of Johann Christian Heinroth (1773–1843), but was nowhere to be found in the otherwise brilliant pioneering work of Charcot, Bernheim, Janet, and other exemplars of the French school.[31] It fell to Freud to give a scientific account of psychological development that showed the stages a primitive primate had to traverse to become a mature human being, in the process recapitulating the whole evolutionary psychological development of the human species. Quite incidentally, he provided a normative definition of maturity that still stands three quarters of a century later. That definition includes the qualities of being active, independent, aware of one's needs, able to see what *is* despite what one wants, and above all, able to work productively and to love others as separate individuals rather than as extensions of oneself.[32]

Most importantly for our understanding of psychopathology, Freud showed that mental illness goes beyond disturbed anatomy and physiology of the brain; more meaningfully, it represents fixations at or regressions to primitive stages in psychological development. Moreover, he showed how maturational pressures can lead to a defensive burying of primitive urges in the unconscious, the deliberate recovery of which is actively resisted by the dynamic unconscious. But the repressed tends to return under its own pressure in the form of neurotic symptoms, reenactments of early relationships, parapraxes, and dream contents. Freud provided a symbology to decode the unconscious meaning of these returns of the repressed.

He also satisfied the human need to recognize a prime mover of the whole human enterprise. Eros (the sexual instinct, broadly interpreted) and, in later writings, the aggressive instinct, both derived from Darwin's theory of evolution, become the driving forces behind human achievement and destruction. These instincts, often operating unconsciously from their base in the subpersonality called the id, to a very great degree control our unexamined and neurotic lives. The purpose of Freudian psychotherapy is to bring the instincts under conscious control: to put ego, as Freud expressed it, where id alone had been.

For this purpose Freud devised a modification of hypnotherapy that induced an altered state of hypersusceptibility to change that did not insult the intelligence or violate the autonomy of the patient. The old-time relationship between hypnotist and subject (or priest and sinner) was obviously authoritarian and impositional, dependent upon a submissive attitude in the subject. Freud's therapy, more in keeping with modern liberal ideals, based its authority not on the position or prestige of the therapist but on the power of his or her insights, on the interpretations provided in penetrating the veils of the unconscious. This is extremely important, because among those most in need of psychotherapy are many who understandably are too independent, skeptical, or plain mistrustful to allow themselves to be put into a hypnotic trance. But to enter into a receptive state of mind in which their critical intelligence is not bypassed, in which they are expected to be active participants in rather than passive recipients of psychological growth—this is another matter entirely. It is, in fact, what the psychoanalytic method promises and frequently delivers.

The emotional neutrality and conversational reserve of the analyst, coupled with hiding his or her facial expressions behind the couch and setting the expectation of uncensored free associations, create a sensory-deprivation situation conducive to the bubbling up of repressed feelings and memories from the unconscious.[33] These contents are then named and explained and, in the process, robbed of their power to influence behavior. The procedure is beautifully designed to recapture forgotten bad experiences from childhood by promoting their reenactment in the therapeutic relationship, affording an opportunity to correct the distortions inherent in the clash of past expectations with current realities.

The rules of the psychoanalytic approach have taught a whole generation of therapists how to discover early formative experiences and to uncover hidden contents in the patient's unconscious while overcoming the sticky hostile-dependent, antitherapeutic feelings that are concurrently aroused. Without the saving grace of psychoanalytic technique, these neurotic attitudes, natural consequences of the focus on intimate feelings and the patient's need to replay old, sick relationships, would completely undermine the therapeutic process.

Adler, Jung, and Rank

The contributions of Jung, Rank, and Adler to modern psychotherapy cannot be considered apart from those of Freud,[34] for each of them developed neglected aspects of psychoanalytic theory and thereby influenced the content of therapy without fundamentally alerting its formal technique, with only a few exceptions. Major technical innovations were left to the contemporary post-Freudians, who were far enough removed from Freud's direct influence to make radical changes in his approach without regard for personal loyalties. It must not be forgotten that Adler, Jung, and Rank, once devoted disciples of Freud, never really transcended his psychoanalytic methods, even though they rejected some of his ideas.

What they had in common was a profound skepticism as to the adequacy of the belief system that Freud offered in place of traditional religion. They felt he underestimated what men live by in according such preeminence to the sexual instinct in human motivation and, even more importantly, to retrospective intellectual analysis in human healing. All three pointed to forces in the personality more meaningful than instinctual expression. They believed that these forces would not achieve creative expression merely through intellectual analysis and conscious insight, that is, by achieving Freud's aim of putting ego where id alone had been.

For Adler, these other forces were the need for social communion (*Gemeinschaftsguefühl*) and the sense of contributing to the betterment of mankind.[35] Adler also pointed to the human need to overcome the sense of physical inferiority, inherent in the human condition but taking specific form in the psychosomatically impaired, as a major personal motivation. In his early writings, he argued that this compensatory striving for superiority typically leads to neurotic life goals and life-styles, characterized by egocentric arrogance and competitiveness.[36] In his later writings, Adler conceived of the striving for superiority as a potentially positive force in the personality that could be directed toward the achievement of social goods.[37]

What is not clear is how Adlerian therapy would promote the constructive expression of these forces other than by an insight-oriented analytic psychotherapy. Adler gives no systematic presentation of his psychotherapeutic technique. What is clearer is that, by his emphasis on the family context and on the importance of social education and action as the way out of self-centered neurosis, Adler is the spiritual father of the social therapies—the group, family, and milieu approaches that have dominated late twentieth-century psychotherapy. More than anyone, he was responsible for the interpersonal, transactional framework on which they depend.

Jung agreed with Adler that neither the meaning nor the cure of neurosis can be contained in a retrospective causal analysis of the individual's past experience, but must involve a prospective synthesis of the individual's future goals.[38] Neurosis, according to Jung, is not all sickness from the past but expresses the individual's aspirations for a higher health in the future. To explain where these higher goal-seeking tendencies come from, Jung rejected Freud's narrow emphasis on the unconscious repressed (the personal unconscious of buried instinctual wishes) and instead outlined his theory of the collective or transpersonal unconscious, a deeper level that contains the more global aspirations of mankind as expressed in our common dreams, myths, fairy tales, and religious legends.[39] Despite the fact that the reader has difficulty in fully grasping Jung's concept of the collective unconscious—what is needed is some account of how memories are stored *between* brains, not just *in* them—the notion, nevertheless, has enormous metaphorical power in providing a bridge between the mental functioning of the individual and the mentalities of larger groups of mankind, such as those responsible for ethnic and national character and the contagious psychology of crowds, which Gustave Le Bon had earlier described.

The nature of the universal tendencies contained in the transpersonal unconscious, which give direction to the instincts, was described by Jung in his theory of the archetypes. These include the soul (*anima* and *animus*), the spirit (*old wise man* and *magna mater*), and most importantly, the self. Jung maintained that deep in the unconscious of every human being resides the archetype of the true self, and the main purpose of life (as well as psychotherapy) is to realize this image, this central program, with all its potentialities, in the individual life as lived in the world. This is achieved by a process that Jung called *individuation*, not to be confused with later uses of the term, which culminates in an integrated self that is creative and beyond purely egocentric concerns. It is clear that for Jung the realization of the self is bound up with discovering the archetype of the God-image within oneself, and thus individuation has a deeply spiritual dimension in Jungian therapy.[40] The extent to which we modern men and women, in search of a soul, can once again meaningfully speak of an image of god will occupy us again in the last chapter.

To Jung's archetypes in the deep unconscious, Otto Rank made an important addition: the prototypes (his word for archetypes) of the hero and the artist.[41] Rank nowhere made it clear that the prototypes reside in the unconscious. Bound up with his rejection of Freud and the Freudian unconscious, Rank did not cast his mature exploration of the depths of the personality in terms of conscious versus unconscious processes. Therefore, what follows is an interpretation of Rank's meaning, influenced by Progoff's important study.[42]

For Rank, becoming a hero or an artist is the acme of human achievement and the only path of healing open to the neurotic, who in Rank's view is defined as an unfulfilled or failed artist-hero, one who is blocked in his or her creative expression. To become creative again the neurotic (according to Rank) must develop an ideology, a belief system, that strengthens his or her will in a creative way. And this belief cannot be derived exclusively from an intellectual, insight-oriented psychotherapy such as Freud's. A psychotherapy dedicated mainly to analytic awareness, to increasing self-consciousness and self-control, is itself a neurotic symptom rather than a cure for neurosis, according to Rank. This is the idea behind Karl Kraus's famous saying that psychoanalysis is the disease for which it purports to be the cure, and Allen Wheelis's admonition that we moderns, in our readiness to put our backs to the couch, sometimes fail to put our shoulders to the wheel.[43]

Heroic acts and artistic creation come from the will, not the intellect, and the blocked creative will requires a strengthening belief to become unblocked. But an analytic psychology can only explain away beliefs and ideologies, not provide vitalizing beliefs of its own. The self-consciousness it promotes can only cast doubt on the creative impulse (which becomes "sicklied over by the pale cast of thought") or tame it to a mere mode of therapeutic self-expression, as in so many of the limp, "psychoanalytic" plays and novels of the post–World War II period. It cannot reach down into the transpersonal, unconscious depths of the soul to create something that goes beyond the merely timely or merely personal confession, that goes beyond individual psychology.[44] As Rank put it in his last written words, "Man is born beyond psychology and he dies beyond it but he can *live* beyond it only through vital experience of his own—in religious terms, through revelation, conversion, or rebirth."[45]

This vital experience is associated with a belief in one's immortality. The will must believe in its own permanence, in the timelessness of its work. The will to immortality culminates in an act of faith that one's lifework will achieve lasting value and that one's personal problems are only part of the struggle inherent in the heroic life of being creative. If the suffering is no longer regarded as "neurotic" but rather as the inevitable pain of being on the rocky, steep path to fulfillment, then the blocked artist will finally cease to be blocked, and his life—in all its expressions—will become a work of art with lasting value. According to Rank, the greatest deficiency of the Freudian worldview derives from its failure to address the necessity of man's believing that he will not come to nothing when he dies. He must believe that he will endure in some form in order to become truly creative. In delivering the death blow to traditional religion, Freud failed to provide the necessary spiritual sustenance that it had once offered.[46]

What are the techniques of the Rankian therapy that will make good on this human need? Such a revelation or conversion experience seems to go beyond psychology and beyond psychotherapy; but surely psychotherapy can prepare the ground for it. Once again, in Rank as in Jung and Adler, one finds indications as to *what* needs to be dealt with in therapy that is different from an analytic approach, but no *how to* that is significantly different, apart from his early emphasis on a time-limited will therapy.[47] For these advances in technique, one must look to the post-Freudians.

Before approaching this contribution of post-Freudian therapists, we must gather together the fruits of our harvest from the history of psychotherapy. Psychotherapy came into being because of the existence of mental suffering.[48] Although mental distress had been thought to derive from some form of alien spirit invasion, it was ultimately seen to derive from the mind's own complex makeup, particularly its proneness to break up into subpersonalities, which tend to operate unconsciously (i.e., outside the awareness of the conscious self).

When a split-off subpersonality operates in harmony with the conscious self, it can serve as a highly positive force in the individual's life, functioning in creative and protective ways. But when it operates in conflict with the conscious self, the result is mental suffering and illness. The cure of such conflict has long been the province of religious healing depending on the ancient practices of prayer, profession, confession, absolution, and exorcism. But with the advent of the Enlightenment in the eighteenth century, it became the province of scientific medicine. In place of an appeal to supernatural forces typified by exorcism, the healing effect was shown to be attainable entirely by naturalistic means, typified by hypnosis. It was demonstrated that under hypnosis, neurotic suffering could be both induced and relieved. It could be induced by implanting a pathogenic idea in a dissociated subpersonality, and it could be relieved by bringing the dissociated subpersonality into awareness and suggesting away its pathogenic ideas.

The major development of modern dynamic psychotherapy has been to remove neurotic suffering by reintegrating the alienated, pathogenic subpersonality without inducing a hypnotic trance. The process is achieved in a nonimpositional manner but in an altered state of hypersuggestible, waking consciousness induced by the sensory-depriving, attention-focusing features of the analytic situation. In this state of enhanced susceptibility to change, the therapeutic process is furthered by a progressive awareness of unconscious motivation. With progressive self-awareness comes progressive self-control, a liberation from primitive and irrational forces so that free, rational choices can be made.

The problem with this process of therapy is that although for some it may be sufficient to dispel neurosis, for others it falls short of providing a healing experience. Among the latter are the artistic-neurotic types who are blocked in their creative expression and who can be healed only by overcoming the blocks. This cannot be achieved solely by resolving conflicts in the unconscious repressed, though this is admittedly an important first step. Rather, the artist-hero must dig more deeply into the creative unconscious to locate and realize the true self. This realization is tantamount to having a revelation experience or, stated less grandly, to being gripped with an undeniable faith in the existence of a higher, unquenchable power within: an inviolable self. To have the fullest possible life, that part of the unconscious containing the creative self must be uncovered and revealed to consciousness, just as the part that contains the instincts must be uncovered. Viktor Frankl had such an uncovering revelation of an inviolable self amidst the life-threatening degradations of the concentration camp.[49] He credited the experience, by virtue of which the ultimate meaning and purpose of life became clear, with his survival and triumph over the dark forces threatening his being and the soul of mankind.

That purpose is to give expression to the timeless universality of the self by creating in external reality one or more enduring works of art, morality, or science. By these creative acts, the creator assures the continued manifestations of the self after biological death and thus achieves a measure of immortality. The question that remains is whether the self can endure as a personal entity. I shall come back to this universal hope, as one always does, at the end of the journey.

The significant developments in post-Freudian therapy take for granted the major discoveries of Freud, Adler, Jung, and Rank. Integrating the divergent viewpoints of these four may require a rounding off of this or that idea (e.g., Freud's psychic determinism or Jung's collective unconscious) but assumes an essential validity to the general thrust of each one's approach. Their viewpoints are regarded as being complementary rather than contradictory. In one way or another, Adler, Jung, and Rank pointed out that in addition to being a psychological being, humans are also spiritual beings—that is, they have existential needs that go beyond being well analyzed and free of symptoms to finding a higher meaning in life. Therefore, a successful psychotherapy in the post-Freudian and postdogmatic religious age must address this "being-need," to use Maslow's term.[50] It must find ways of helping predisposed human beings tap into the spiritual deep springs of the creative unconscious. Formulating such an approach is the purpose of this book. The developments in the sciences and in Western culture on which it depends will now be briefly reviewed.

THE ARTIST-THERAPIST

The most important of these developments is a phenomenon in the field of psychotherapy itself: the emergence of the post-Freudian artist-therapist. What I mean by this appelation is a psychotherapist, less an intellectual or scientist then an intuitive artist, who cannot comfortably fit into any orthodoxy or school. Yet he or she has learned from Freud and the other depth psychologists how the unconscious works and what the basic rules of dynamic therapy are, even if he or she takes liberties with them to realize a personal artistic vision. For such a therapist, Freud's discoveries are both taken for granted and transcended; therefore, instead of antianalytic or nonanalytic, he or she is most accurately described as postanalytic or post-Freudian.

The prototype of the postanalytic therapist was Sandor Ferenczi, a Hungarian psychiatrist who died in 1933. Ferenczi was perhaps the most gifted therapist of Freud's inner circle, not a great theoretician but a natural healer who was irrepressibly innovative and artistic in his methods.[51] Predictably, as the psychoanalytic approach became increasingly formalized, Ferenczi got into trouble with other analysts and finally Freud himself for his "wild analysis." What he recognized was that some neurotics are not so much in conflict as a result of bad experiences as they are simply bereft of good experiences. Instead of having conflicts needing analysis, they had love-lacks needing filling. So Ferenczi quite naturally tried to fill the emptiness by providing the experiences his patients had missed out on because of inadequate parenting. He reputedly held them on his lap and talked to them like hurt children. Put in its simplest terms, he gave them caring affection at a time when therapists were mainly giving interpretations. He was one of the first interactive therapists and served as the inspiration for the more active artist-therapists who came after him, such as Sechéhaye, Rosen, Moreno, and Milton Erickson.[52]

What these first post-Freudians shared in common was an ability to intuit directly the patient's unconscious feelings and needs and to provide the love, direction, and confrontation—the actual experiences, not just the explanations—necessary to allaying them. In doing this, the psychotherapist was reverting to type, becoming an active doer rather than just a source of insights, once more laying claim to the mantle of hypnotist, actor, or (in Moreno's psychodrama) director. But their use of direction and suggestion, in contrast to that of the hypnotists of an earlier day, was psychodynamically informed and therefore designed to meet and give expression to the patient's needs rather than impose on them.

It has been my privilege to observe at first hand the work of several artist-therapists of the early post-Freudian era. The first, Elvin Semrad, interviewed patients in front of my classes at Harvard Medical School in the 1950s. Although labeled an orthodox Freudian, he was one of a kind and strictly unclassifiable. What Semrad did supremely well was to talk in public with patients about their innermost, private feelings. He did this in front of a crowd of medical students, psychiatry residents, psychologists, nurses, and social workers, a group of strangers who hardly deserved to hear such confidences. But we learned to watch and listen and, in the process, became worthier recipients of these private revelations.

I once witnessed his suggesting to an agoraphobic woman that she experienced a wide range of lurid sensations in her genitals whenever she went out on the street. The woman kept exclaiming, "But, Dr. Semrad, this is uncanny! How do you know these things?" Both she and we became increasingly amazed with each new revelation about the state of her vaginal sensations and her wish to be a whore. When the interview was over, Semrad pointed out that he had just performed major psychosurgery. Every one of us believed it, for we had sensations in the backs of our necks, no less uncanny than the ones in the patient's vagina, to prove it. We were certain that the patient would never be the same again, nor would we. In later years I developed reservations about the value of such public exposures, but there was no denying that Semrad did it with great artistry.

Carl Whitaker, a colleague at the University of Wisconsin in the late 1960s and early 1970s, was a master at telling the therapeutic tale or parable, typically involving purported experiences of his own. The parable, often told within minutes of starting the interview, accomplished several things at once. It established empathic connection with the patient's unconscious wishes and fears and validated their existence. Moreover, it seemed to say that the therapist had similar feelings and had made peace with them. The story also suggested what the causes of such troubles might be and how they could be resolved. Often, they simply had to be seen as absurd and undeserving of serious attention.

For example, a young man of ambiguous sexuality complained to Whitaker of problems in getting ahead in his work. Without so much as mentioning the patient's obvious concerns about his sexuality, Whitaker, sounding somewhat androgynous himself, launched into a story about his sexual feelings for another man and how he wanted to have breasts, including what he had done to grow them. At some point during this travesty the patient became annoyed at Whitaker and said he would like to kick him. Whitaker answered, "Why don't you?" No sooner had the patient tapped him lightly with his foot than Whitaker kicked him back harder and asked if he would like to do it again. They traded kicks a couple more times, and then the patient got up, said thank you, and left. No direct mention was made of any of the issues dealt with: the fear of aggressive and competitive feelings toward men, the envy of women, the fear of homosexuality and the importance for a man to accept his feminine self, all of which were germane to this patient's troubles and had been magically addressed in this bizarre encounter.

Both Semrad and Whitaker were showmen, and their work was often highly dramatic. But this is not an essential feature of post-Freudian experiential therapy. The point is illustrated by the work of two Philadelphia colleagues, Salvador Minuchin and Robert Pottash. Minuchin, a family therapist whom I observed at the Philadelphia Child Guidance Clinic in the late 1970s, is an artist at giving dynamically informed directives that, if carried out, will effect significant change in both individual and family systems.[53] In seeing a family with a depressed adolescent daughter who is much too involved with her father, Minuchin asked the father to turn over completely the care of the daughter to the mother, confining his efforts solely to supporting the mother in this task. In getting the family to comply with this directive, Minuchin effectively extricated the daughter from the triangle between her parents and forced the parents to deal directly with their long-standing conflict with each other that had led to the unhealthy father-daughter relationship. The artistry here lay in translating interlocking personal dynamics into family structural terms and then being able to modify those structures suggestively.

Similarly, in telling a wildly rebellious teenage boy that his parents have let him down by providing few limits on his behavior, Minuchin redefined the whole meaning of the symptomatic behavior, reallocating some of the blame and responsibility. If the boy accepts the redefinition, then Minuchin has gained great leverage in getting him to change, provided that the parents do their part. If they do, then the boy must either change or define himself as oppositional or out of control. If he acquiesces, then everyone in the family will have been affected both internally and behaviorally. In all this, no mention is made of inner motives and unconscious needs and wishes, the usual psychodynamic interpretations. Yet, Minuchin's interventions are informed by an exquisite understanding of these forces.

Robert Pottash, who also taught at Philadelphia's Child Guidance Clinic, is a master of therapeutic karate. He delivers psychological blows that shatter patients' defenses and readies them for personality change. Rather than a "headshrinker," Pottash would more accurately be described as a "nutcracker." His methods are sensible but powerfully penetrating. For example, the traditional therapist usually accepts the patient's expressions of anger toward him as a good thing. He will ask the whys and wherefores of it but will end up affirming its value as a self-assertion. In contrast, Pottash might counterattack, arguing that his response is more faithful to reality and more stimulating of growth. If you express your anger toward authority figures out in the world, you will probably end up being penalized or even fired. So it is not always such a good thing for the therapist to encourage self-expression indiscriminately. The old Mafia percept, "Don't get angry, get even," is closer to the mark but too petty. Pottash's approach seems to say, "Don't get angry, get it done."

For example, a patient accused Pottash of a monetary motive in suggesting that he come twice instead of once each week. Pottash responded that such an accusation was personally offensive. Furthermore, he could not understand why the patient would be willing to work with a therapist whom he thought capable of such an action. Needless to say, there was no question of increasing the frequency of sessions after that, yet the issue continued to exert a powerful and beneficial effect on the subsequent course of therapy. The intervention raised questions about the basis of all intimate relationships and when they ought to be terminated.

There is an obvious element of harshness in this approach. To promote change, the therapist implicitly threatens the continuity of the relationship. This is an intimidating deployment of personal power that, given the patient's dependent position, is hardly a fair way to fight. But it issues an effective demand to the patient to transform primitive anger into more maturely effective forms of aggression.

What Ferenczi, Minuchin, and the other post-Freudians share in common is a diminished estimate of the value of intellectual interpretations in doing therapy. Instead of stating the contents of an interpretation, they provide the corrective emotional experience, to use Franz Alexander's phrase, that such an interpretation would dictate but cannot itself provide.[54] This might involve a show of interest or affection, a giving of direction, a rap on the knuckles, or a talking to the patient's unconscious in a language that it can understand. As the reader will see in subsequent chapters, these post-Freudian methods and later innovations in biological, behavioral, family, and group interventions make it possible to achieve the broader aims of the bio-existential therapist, who puts his or her values on the line instead of proclaiming moral neutrality.

THE POSTMATERIALIST PERSPECTIVE

But it is begging the question somewhat to account for the emergence of a post-Freudian therapy by the appearance of post-Freudian therapists. The question being begged is *why* this new breed of therapists appeared. One obvious reason is that Freud had come along before them, permitting them to stand on his broad shoulders and thereby to see farther than he himself had seen. The importance of this factor cannot be overestimated. But there is a gulf between Freud and the post-Freudians that no amount of shoulder straddling can explain. Reading Freud is to take a cold bath in rational thought. The post-Freudians have a more intense spiritual dimension that transcends intellectual analysis without denying its value. This dimension is hard to find in Freud. Bettelheim, in his book *Freud and Man's Soul,* argues that the antispiritual flavor of his writings does not appear in the original German but only in its poor English translation.[55] But considering the closeness to Freud and the expertise of those involved in the official translation,[56] one has difficulty avoiding the conclusion that his writings easily lend themselves to such "distortion."

A less torturous interpretation is that Freud's theory bears the imprint of the mechanistic scientific worldview, derived from Newton, Darwin, and Helmholtz, current in his time. At the very moment Freud was making his creative synthesis of the medical psychology and evolutionary biology of the late nineteenth century, however, its undergirding scientific structure was undergoing revolutionary changes. Einstein was formulating his theories of relativity and clearing the way for quantum physics. This new physics fundamentally alters our conceptions of reality and causation—so much so that, from its perspective, Freud's ideas about instinctual and psychic determinism apply only within narrowly circumscribed conditions of observation. There are, in fact, multiple perspectives, complementary to each other rather than contradictory, that must be taken together to provide a broader truth about human motivation.

What the new physics does is put the mind back into nature, from which it had been abstracted to create the body of materialistic science. With Einstein, science reached the limit of what it can know without taking account of the act of knowing (i.e., without becoming self-conscious). Once this is done, science has to transcend its own materialism, because it sees that matter, space, time, and causality—the fundamental facts of scientific knowledge—are mental constructs, as Kant first convincingly showed. They have no absolute reality but instead are relative to the properties of the observing mind.

What this leads to is a profoundly postmaterialistic view of the world. As Sir James Jeans put it, "the universe begins to look more like a great thought than a great machine."[57] In the same spirit, Eddington maintained, "The stuff of the world is mind-stuff"[58]—not material stuff. Paul Davies, the leading contemporary interpreter of the new physics, points out that its worldview is in "closer accord with mysticism than materialism."[59] One has only to acquaint oneself with some of the immaterial properties of cosmology and particle physics to begin to appreciate the point. The "anthropic principle," which maintains that the universe exists in its present form, full of astonishing uniformities, so that intelligent observers can come into existence to witness it, is only one striking expression of this theoretical trend.[60] Instead of regarding the discoveries of Copernicus, Darwin, and Freud as three great blows to man's narcissism (a typically Freudian interpretation[61]), the new physics might characterize them as three heavy drumbeats of the human mind's relentless march away from petty grandiosity toward the true grandeur of a universal perspective.

But what has all this to do with psychotherapy? It justifies a different approach to explanation and treatment of mental illness. From this viewpoint, there is no one cause of a mental symptom, and therefore no single intervention. Instead, there are multiple determinants: as many as there are human perspectives, and each with a limited sphere of applicability. There is no longer any justification for giving priority to physical-mechanical explanations and interventions, except to achieve specific pragmatic objectives. On this view, depression can represent a problem with chemistry, instincts, self-concept, social network, and values. Each of these levels of explanation fits on an endless hierarchical loop,[62] each of which constitutes a valid but circumscribed viewpoint.

Causation, in this scheme, represents multiple interactions; all the variables can work together to create depression, and every level can interact with every other level. For instance, changing one's chemistry may end up changing one's values, but changing one's values may end up changing one's chemistry, self-concept, or friendships. From this quantum perspective, the therapist cannot afford to neglect the patient's beliefs, ideals, or aesthetic and moral values in understanding his or her suffering or in trying to heal it. Nor can the therapist neglect the patient's chemistry or psychology. Yet, this is a scientific worldview that goes beyond chemistry and beyond psychology. It is distinctively postmaterialist and post-Freudian.

The third major development leading to a post-Freudian psychotherapy has been the discovery of effective psychoactive chemicals and the enhanced understanding of mental and neural functioning made possible by their utilization.[63] This development has two parts. In the first one, the stabilizers of mood and cognition now available have not only emptied the mental hospitals but made it possible for suffering human beings to divert their psychic energies to higher concerns than fighting off depression or paranoia. Used adjunctively with psychotherapy, the chemicals can facilitate the process and elevate the goals to a realm beyond psychological symptom relief, as we shall see in the chapters ahead.

The second part has been the widespread experimentation with "mind-expanding" chemicals that began in the 1960s. With LSD and other hallucinogens, chemical adjuncts have been found that can facilitate the journey into the archetypal core of the deep unconscious.[64] Unfortunately, the effects have often been disastrous, for in that core resides the common "mythic stuff" not only of art and religion but also of psychosis. The possibility of better psychedelics with fewer harmful side effects and their utilization only in properly prepared subjects under expert supervision hold out hope for a marked advance in treating mental distress and advancing human consciousness as a whole.

Finally, in recent years, behavioral scientists have been developing a true psychology of consciousness and its altered states.[65] This has both a technical side and an existential face. In its technical aspect, important work has been done in cerebral lateralization via split-brain preparations. As a result, many of the features of primary process thinking, characteristic of the Freudian unconscious, have been located in the nondominant hemisphere of the brain.[66] This work has spurred a renewed scientific interest in the method and language of change[67]: the focusing of consciousness and the hypnotic patter addressed to the right brain and capable of invoking and influencing its change-producing processes.

In its spiritual, existential aspect, we have witnessed during the past half century the diffusion into the West of Eastern mystical ideas and practices.[68] We owe to some of these mystical ideas, particularly to Hasidism's experientialism and Sufism's doctrine of the evolution of consciousness, a hospitable environment for a psychotherapy committed to a never-ending spiritual growth.

This is the most important psychological development of our time: the realization that we as individuals, as patients and therapists, are capable of continuous psychological development. The evolution of our consciousness until we taste the infinity of its means is the true purpose of our life and the highest goal of our work. It is becoming our self.

NOTES

1. Jerome Frank, *Persuasion and Healing,* Baltimore: Johns Hopkins Press, 1961.
2. Ibid., pp. 2–3.
3. William Sargant, *Battle for the Mind,* New York: Doubleday, 1957; J. Murphy, "Psychotherapeutic Aspects of Shamanism on St. Lawrence Island, Alaska," in Ari Kiev, ed., *Magic, Faith, and Healing,* New York: Free Press, 1964, pp. 53–83; Henri Ellenberger, *The Discovery of the Unconscious,* New York: Basic Books, 1970, pp. 3–52.
4. Frank, op. cit., pp. 36–64.
5. Idries Shah, in his illuminating work, *The Sufis* (Garden City, NY: Doubleday, 1964, pp. 58–59), attributes Freud's sexual theories to El-Ghazali of Persia (1058–1111) and Jung's archetypal theory to Ibn El-Arabi (b. 1164), both sages of the Islamic faith. Similarly, David Bakan, in his *Sigmund Freud and the Jewish Mystical tradition* (New York: Schocken, 1958) attributes many of Freud's ideas (e.g., man's innate bisexuality, the methods of free association and symbol interpretation) to the Kabbalah.
6. M. L. Smith, G. Glass, and T. Miller, *The Benefits of Psychotherapy,* Baltimore: Johns Hopkins, 1980. What this massive review fails to establish is that some forms of psychotherapy are better than others.
7. Ellenberger, op. cit.
8. Gregory Zilboorg, *A History of Medical Psychology,* New York: Norton, 1941.
9. George Mora, Historical and Theoretical Trends in Psychiatry. In H. I. Kaplan, A. M. Freedman, and B. J. Sadock, eds., *Comprehensive Textbook of Psychiatry,* 3rd ed., Baltimore: Williams and Wilkins, 1980.
10. Ibid., p. 45.
11. J. Sprenger, and H. Kramer, *Malleus Maleficarum,* London: Rodker, 1928.
12. J. Weyer, *De Praestigiis Daemonum,* Amsterdam: Bonset, 1967.
13. Zilboorg, op. cit., p. 200.
14. Ellenberger, op. cit., pp. 58–59.
15. Ibid., p. 72.
16. Ibid., p. 74–83.
17. Ibid., pp. 126–141.
18. Zilboorg, op. cit., pp. 362–363.
19. Ibid., p. 485.
20. Ibid., p. 364.
21. Ellenberger, op. cit., pp. 406–409.
22. Ibid., pp. 377–386.
23. Ibid., pp. 312–313.

24. F. W. H. Myers, *Human Personality and Its Survival of Bodily Death*, London: Longman, Green, 1903.
25. Ellenberger, op. cit., pp. 145–147.
26. Ibid., pp. 314–315.
27. Ibid., pp. 315–317.
28. R. Assagioli, *Psychosynthesis*, New York: Viking, 1965.
29. A. Schopenhauer, *The World as Will and Representation*, New York: Dover, 1969.
30. Ellenberger, op. cit., pp. 236–237.
31. Mora, op. cit., p. 65.
32. S. Freud, *The Standard Edition of the Complete Psychological Works*, 24 vols., London: Hogarth Press, 1960.
33. D. Rapaport, "The Theory of Ego Autonomy." In M. Gill, ed., *The Collected Papers of David Rapaport*, New York: Basic Books, 1967.
34. Ira Progoff, *The Death and Rebirth of Psychology*, New York: McGraw-Hill, 1956.
35. Alfred Adler, *Understanding Human Nature*, New York: Garden City, 1927.
36. Alfred Adler, *The Neurotic Constitution*, New York: Moffat, Yard, 1917.
37. Alfred Adler, *Social Interest: A Challenge to Mankind*, London: Faber and Faber, 1938.
38. Carl Jung, *Symbols of Transformation*, New York: Pantheon, 1956.
39. Carl Jung, *The Archetypes and the Collective Unconscious*, Princeton, New Jersey: Princeton University Press, 1969.
40. Progoff, op. cit., pp. 177–187; Ellenberger, op. cit., p. 725.
41. Otto Rank, *Art and Artist*, New York: Knopf, 1932.
42. Progoff, op. cit., pp. 188–253.
43. A. Wheelis, "Will and Psychoanalysis," *J. Amer. Psychoanalytic Assoc.* 4:285–303, 1956.
44. Otto Rank, *Beyond Psychology*, New York: Dover, 1958.
45. Ibid., p. 16.
46. Otto Rank, *Psychology and the Soul*, New York: A. S. Barnes, 1961.
47. Otto Rank, *Will Therapy* and *Truth and Reality*, New York: Knopf, 1945.
48. The existence of mental pain, along with the existence of art and religion, is regarded by Evelyn Underhill as one of the central mysteries of human life. In her book, *Mysticism* (New York: Dutton, 1961), she makes a convincing case that none of them furthers any material purposes, only spiritual ones.
49. Victor Frankl, *Man's Search for Meaning*, New York, Simon and Schuster, 1984.
50. A. Maslow, *The Farther Reaches of Human Nature*, New York: Viking, 1971.
51. S. Ferenczi, *Final Contributions to the Problems and Methods of Psychoanalysis*, London: Hogarth Press, 1955.
52. An overview of the work of these pioneering active therapists can be found in David Greenwald's edited volume, *Active Psychotherapy* (New York: Atherton Press, 1967). Of particular interest is Milton Erickson's work, which has been described in a lively fashion by Jay Haley in *Uncommon Therapy* (New York: Norton, 1973) and presented in his edited volume of selected papers by Erickson, *Advanced Techniques of Hypnosis and Therapy* (New York: Grune and Stratton, 1967).
53. S. Minuchin, *Families and Family Therapy*, Cambridge, Massachusetts: Harvard University Press, 1974. I am unaware of any publications that adequately describe the mature clinical work of Semrad, Whitaker, or Pottash. Each has taught a great deal in public seminars or workshops, however, and an extensive videotape library of Minuchin and Whitaker's work can be found in the Philadelphia Child Guidance Clinic Library.
54. F. Alexander and T. French, *Psychoanalytic Therapy*, New York: Ronald Press, 1946.
55. B. Bettelheim, *Freud and Man's Soul*, New York: Alfred A. Knopf, 1983.

56. Freud, op. cit. The translations were made by James Strachey in collaboration with Anna Freud, Alix Strachey, and Alan Tyson. In addition, Strachey acknowledges the work of the "Psychoanalytic Glossary Committee" headed by Ernest Jones and extensive correspondence with Kurt Eissler. In her preface to Volume 24, Anna Freud is lavish in her praise of Strachey's "scholarly precision."
57. Sir James Jeans, *The Mysterious Universe,* Cambridge, England: Cambridge University Press, 1937.
58. A. S. Eddington, *The Philosophy of Physical Science,* Cambridge, England: Cambridge University Press, 1939.
59. P. Davies, *God and the New Physics,* New York: Simon and Schuster, 1983, p. vii.
60. P. Davies, *The Accidental Universe,* Cambridge, England: Cambridge University Press, 1982.
61. Freud, op. cit., Vol. XVII, pp. 139–143. This is Freud's most developed account of the three blows to man's narcissism brought about by modern science: Copernicus's discovery that this planet, Earth, is not the center of the universe; Darwin's demonstration that his species is not something more special than an evolved animal; and Freud's own marshaling of evidence that man's conscious mind is not in complete control of his actions. It is characteristic of Freud's pessimistic outlook to emphasize the deprecatory aspects of these great achievements rather than their liberating, expansive influence.
62. D. R. Hofstader, *Gödel, Escher, Bach,* New York: Vintage, 1980. The author presents a fascinating discussion of strange hierarchical loops that account for some of the paradoxical attributes of mind.
63. A good popular survey of the state of psychopharmacology can be found in P. Wender and D. Klein, *Mind, Mood, and Medicine,* New York: New American Library, 1981. The authors seem to regard psychotherapy as an adjunct to the drug therapy of psychiatric symptoms, hardly of equal, much less of greater, importance.
64. L. Grinspoon and J. Bakalar, "Drug Dependence: Non-Narcotic Agents," in Kaplan, Freedman, and Sadock: *Comprehensive Textbook of Psychiatry,* op. cit., pp. 1614–1629. This is an excellent, brief review of the current state of our knowledge of the psychedelics and the so-called minor drugs of abuse.
65. R. Ornstein, *The Psychology of Consciousness,* New York: Viking, 1972. Also C. Tart, ed., *Altered States of Consciousness,* New York: John Wiley, 1969. In the latter volume, Ludwig's discussion of the characteristics of altered states is particularly fine, as is his appreciation that psychotherapeutic change always involves the induction of an altered state.
66. R. Ornstein, ed., *The Nature of Human Consciousness,* New York: Viking, 1973. See particularly the articles by Gazzaniga and Bogen on lateralization.
67. P. Watzlawick, *The Language of Change,* New York: Basic Books, 1978.
68. These mystical ideas derive from Hasidism, an eastern European adaptation of Kabbalistic teachings and ably presented in Elie Wiesel's *Souls on Fire* (New York: Random House, 1972); Sufism, as presented by Idries Shah in *The Sufis* (New York: Doubleday, 1964); and Zen Buddhism, as presented by D. T. Suzuki in his many works and particularly in his *Zen and Japanese Culture* (New York: Pantheon, 1959).

CHAPTER 3

The Five Modern Schools of Mental Treatment

In reviewing the history of dynamic psychotherapy in the last chapter, I distinguished a pre-Freudian hypnotherapy phase, a Freudian analytic phase, and a post-Freudian existential phase. During the Freudian phase, the emergence of the dissident thinking of Adler, Jung, and Rank recast the meaning of psychopathology and the goals of treatment. In so doing it prepared the way for our contemporary post-Freudian approach, which is less intellectually analytic and more spiritually integrative or ideal seeking. While valuing the Freudian aim of achieving conflict-free maturity, post-Freudian therapy aims beyond psychological adaptation to achieve freedom and creativity, the pinnacles of human achievement.

This way of describing the history, however, makes it sound as if most modern therapists have safely made the transition from a sectarian allegiance to one particular school of thought to a nonsectarian, integrated approach. This is more the exception than the rule. What we still find is a Babel of competing theories, each of which provides only a partial account of mental suffering. In addition to Freudian psychoanalysis and Jungian analytic psychology, we find schools of transactional analysis, cognitive and behavior therapy, primal scream, bioenergetics, gestalt therapy, sensitivity training, structural and strategic family therapy, encounter groups, psychosynthesis, and rational emotive therapy, to give only a partial listing of the different approaches.[1] And as if the field were not fragmented enough, the observer notes on its fringes a scattering of therapeutic cults ranging from relatively benign to clearly dangerous.

Though chaotic, this profusion of therapies has its healthy side. It attests to great ferment within the field, a willingness on the part of practitioners to experiment with new methods rather than cling to old ways. In the history of scientific progress, such chaos is often the prelude to the development of a new paradigm that brings healing and fruitful order to a field.[2] The situation in medicine at the end of last century serves as an instructive example. At that time there existed numerous competing schools of medical treatment. There were homeopathic, osteopathic, eclectic, physiomedical, and allopathic physicians, to name the most prominent varieties. By the 1920s, however, a great pulling together had occurred, and modern medicine emerged from its prescientific adolescence to assume its adult identity.[3] We find ourselves in a similar developmental stage in the field of psychotherapy—a chaotic ego diffusion ripe for an integrative ordering.

In pursuing this analogy to medicine, I would suggest that the multiplicity of approaches in contemporary psychotherapy can be regarded as offshoots of five main schools of mental treatment: the psychodynamic, existential, biomedical, learning theory, and social system approaches. No doubt there is considerable overlap among them, and the situation is further complicated by the dual or even triple percentage of some. For example, one finds in transactional analysis elements of both the psychodynamic and learning theory traditions, and in gestalt therapy elements of the psychodynamic and the existential approaches. Despite (or even because of) these blurrings, the competing schools need to be definitively reconciled and integrated. Providing a schema for doing this is the purpose of the following discussion.

The reason the five traditions have to be integrated is that each of them alone provides an incomplete view of treatment and a partial account of the main etiological factors. Consequently, to offer effective, comprehensive care in the field, the therapist must be able to combine the various approaches. In this task, however, he or she gets very little outside help. For one reason, the proponents of the separate schools present their viewpoints in competitive, monopolistic terms that discourage the free flow of ideas. More ecumenical theorists, on the other hand, rarely attempt to combine more than two of the different approaches, giving the student the idea that the others are not worth serious study.

My aim here is to rise above this parochialism to present the main tenets of each school with objectivity and appreciation. I will try to give each a form that will permit it to be joined together with the others. This will entail some pruning of tenets that would preclude integration: for example, learning theory's rejection of the concepts of diagnosis and disease, which violates the spirit of the biomedical school and also fits poorly with the psychodynamic approach. After offering these formulations, I will propose a pluralistic model for synthesizing the separate schools into the comprehensive bio-existential approach.[4]

THE PSYCHODYNAMIC SCHOOL

The most pervasive and venerable school or tradition is the psychodynamic one, which encompasses the various forms of psychoanalytic psychotherapy ranging from orthodox psychoanalysis itself to the most liberal forms of analytic therapy. Because I have already described its fundamental tenets in the account of Freud's contribution in Chapter 2 and because it is by far the best-known theory of psychotherapy, my discussion here will be brief. To recapitulate, the psychodynamic approach regards neurosis as the pathology of arrested psychological development. This arrest is typically precipitated by anxiety generated by unconscious conflicts between the individual's drives and the strictures of his or her ego and superego. The conflicts, usually originating in childhood, tend to be reenacted throughout the individual's entire life, giving a flavor of predestination to its course. Analytic therapy is devoted to gaining conscious awareness of the previously unconscious conflicts, thereby resolving them, stopping their rigid reliving, and starting up the process of forward psychological development again. In this tradition, then, neurosis is the pathology of immaturity, whereas therapy is the retrospective analysis of its unconscious sources. The approach has its greatest utility in taming primitive drives, bringing them under rational, social control. It can also be effective in summoning forth previously unconscious, destructive subpersonalities and integrating them into a unified self.

THE EXISTENTIAL SCHOOL

The existential tradition derives in part from Adler, Jung, and Rank's critique of psychoanalysis and in part from trends in European thought having their origins in the work of Kierkegaard, Nietzsche, and Husserl, among others. It has achieved its most articulate expression in May, Angel, and Ellenberger's volume of readings, *Existence,* and Irvin Yalom's *Existential Psychotherapy.*[5] The approach also has connections with the human potential movement and what has been called the "third force" of humanistic psychology, typified by the work of Maslow and Rogers.[6] More an attitude toward suffering human beings than merely a technique for treating them, the existential orientation seeks to understand the patient from within his or her own world, that is, from the inner perspective of the subjective sufferer rather than from the outer one of the objective observer. When this point of view is taken, the patient's neurosis is no longer seen as exclusively pathological. Rather, it is also appreciated as the expression of a creative aim—to realize the true self and its ideals.

And what are these ideals? According to Yalom, the main existential concerns of man are achieving freedom and responsibility, finding meaning in life, and facing with dignity one's essential aloneness in the world and the inevitability of one's death. The response to these existential dilemmas defines the highest ideals of the true self. Existential individuals strive to become free by transcending their social conditioning. They attempt to overcome the painful inevitability of death by making a lasting contribution to the living. They find meaning in life by their never-ending quest to develop their self-awareness and their potential.

The greatest potential of such individuals is the capacity to expand their consciousness in such a way that they become creative. First they learn to achieve intimacy with another individual, thereby overcoming personal aloneness. Then they learn increasingly to achieve union with a higher consciousness (the true self), thereby overcoming metaphysical aloneness. In the process, they link up with the whole and tap into its creative reservoir. Freedom, meaning, and passion coalesce to yield creativity. In Rank's view, this is most fully realized in the artist-hero, who dares to defy conventional truth to create a higher vision of truth.

From this perspective, the neurotic symptom represents a temporary strategic retreat to avoid a permanent forfeit of the creative spark. Becoming depressed or detached, truant, or compliant serves to protect the creative will while manifesting the suffering of its blocked expression. The existential sufferer concedes psychological health to avoid forfeiting his or her core integrity of spirit. He or she splits temporarily in order not to become permanently blunted. Whereas in the psychodynamic tradition neurosis represents an arrest at or retreat to the primitive past, in the existential tradition it is the blocked artist's preservation of a creative future. Whereas psychodynamic therapy is a retrospective analysis in the service of achieving ego control, existential therapy is a prospective synthesis in the service of achieving values and beliefs that are activating. The difference is between control and creativity; one should value both without trying to make a life out of either alone. The following case illustrates some of the differences between the two approaches.

Amanda was a 27-year-old mousy librarian who consulted me because of depression. In addition to having both eating and sleep disorders, she felt too socially incompetent and disorganized to go through with her projected marriage. At age 20, she had become sexually promiscuous and then pregnant shortly after her medical missionary father had to be committed to a mental hospital. Taken to a minister in her father's church, Amanda was admonished for her sins and urged to pray for forgiveness. From that day on she never again set foot in a church or prayed to God. Not only did God cease to exist but also the values based, in her mind, on the Judeo-Christian religion. She became exclusively pleasure seeking, a self-professed cynic and hedonist.

She was able to take in my (psychodynamic) interpretations that her promiscuity and subsequent hedonism represented a self-destructive acting out of her anger and disillusionment with her father and the religious ideals he stood for. Unfortunately, she also periodically used these interpretations to torture herself in a self-accusatory manner, taking them as further evidences of her worthlessness. This tendency to criticize herself harshly was similarly traced to her identification with her father's demeaning attitude throughout her childhood and adolescence and with her mother's depression and stern religiosity. Understanding these determinants of her behavior helped her curb their blatant expression but was less effective in helping her come to love herself.

Accomplishing the latter involved a more existential approach. Amanda was helped to see that her promiscuity was not only an angry, rebellious acting out but also an expression of a higher integrity. It represented a refusal to sacrifice her sensuality on the altar of rectitude. By sleeping around, she averted the dried-up, lonely fate that befell her pious mother and younger sister. Given credit for the spirit-conserving function of her neurotic behavior, she began to pepper her previously self-deprecatory talk with remarks like, "Hey, I'm pretty smart and more sensual and artistic than the average person." And she was able ultimately to get married and to emerge as an imaginative, fulfilled human being. She developed many interests and talents and, according to fellow group members, decorated her home with great flair. In time she overcame her disillusionment and regained her belief in the existence of universal values, this time on adult terms.

A standard psychodynamic approach, regarding her acting out as a harkening back to the primitive past, proved to be of only partial value in this case. To think of her as merely sexually acting out missed the constructive, health-seeking purpose of her behavior, the deep-lying integrity and artistic spirit that insisted upon the survival of her sensuality and creativity even in a disguised and degraded form. The appreciation of the positive aspects of neurotic and borderline symptoms, the expression of integrity intrinsic to them, falls within the domain of the existential tradition. Recognizing this aspect of symptoms is also highly supportive; it allows us to affirm what is truly unique and wonderful about our patients.

THE BIOMEDICAL SCHOOL

In the last chapter, I suggested that modern psychotherapy, particularly in its psychodynamic and existential forms, is the offspring of religious faith healing. The crucial difference is that healing is now achieved by faith in the truths of psychology rather than those of theology. The other parent of modern psychotherapy is scientific medicine, and this influence is most apparent in the biomedical approach, which is technological rather than psychological and artistic. It seeks predictability and reproducibility in stamping out mental disease, whereas the more artistically oriented existential approach seeks unpredictability by unleashing in people unique creative forces.

As with the faith-derived psychotherapy traditions, the biomedical approach can trace its origins to antiquity. The ancient Greek physicians knew of depression, hysteria, and other categories of mental illness, but the great advances came in the nineteenth and twentieth centuries with the flowering of the clinical case study in psychiatry. Having barely mentioned medical psychiatry and its approach to mental treatment in the last chapter, I must now give an overview of its major achievements,[7] which are currently having a revolutionary impact on mental treatment.

In the last half of the nineteenth century in France, Falret and Baillarger gave the first adequate clinical descriptions of manic-depressive disease, and Lasègue and Falret of *folie à deux.* Lasègue also described delusions of persecution. Morel outlined the process of the deterioration of mental traits that culminated in premature dementia or, as it came to be called, dementia praecox. At roughly the same time in Germany, Griesinger, the first full-time academic psychiatrist, argued successfully that mental diseases are all brain diseases—disorders of brain chemistry and physiology. Westphal gave a clear description of obsessional thinking, Kahlbaum elucidated the syndrome of catatonia, and Hecker described hebephrenia. Freud's teacher, Meynert, described the hierarchical relationship of cortical and subcortical structures, paving the way for a conception of mental illness as a neurological release phenomenon (i.e., as an escape of primitive subcortical functioning from higher cortical inhibition), an idea that has informed all subsequent psychobiological thinking. Wernicke localized various mental functions in specific areas of the brain and, along with Korsakoff, described the syndrome of alcoholic degeneration. Krafft-Ebing catalogued the manifold syndromes of sexual dysfunction.

Then, at the turn of the century, Emil Kraepelin pulled together these various strands of knowledge to create our modern nosology of mental illness. He distinguished the two major psychoses, dementia praecox (what Bleuler was later to call schizophrenia) and manic-depressive disease. He collected clinical data to show that most schizophrenics follow a deteriorating course, whereas manic-depressives have a waxing and waning course with a return to prepsychotic levels of functioning between exacerbations of the illness. Kraepellin's work was the crowning achievement of this age of mental diagnostics, paving the way for the dawning age of mental therapeutics that was to characterize psychiatry in the twentieth century.

Progress in the medical therapeutics of mental illness has come in ever larger waves throughout our century.[8] Noguchi and Moore discovered the *Treponema pallidum* spirochete as the cause of central nervous system syphilis in 1913, and Wagner-Jauregg introduced the first medically effective treatment for any psychiatric disorder, the malaria therapy of syphilitic insanity, in 1917. In the 1920s Goldberger ascertained the cause of pellagra psychosis to be a nutritional deficiency in need of dietary treatment. Then, between 1935 and 1937, Sakel introduced insulin coma treatment for schizophrenia; Meduna discovered convulsive treatment, subsequently shown to be highly effective for depression and mania in its electrically induced form (as developed by Cerletti and Bini); Moniz ushered in the field of psychosurgery and showed that prefrontal lobotomy was effective in ameliorating some cases of intractable compulsive and bizarre behaviors; and Bradley introduced the paradoxical use of amphetamines for hyperactive children.

Finally, between 1949 and the mid-1960s, the psychoactive drugs entered the arena to change psychiatry from a field of relative therapeutic nihilism to one of great optimism. Cade discovered the effects of lithium on manic symptoms, and subsequently Baastrup and Schou demonstrated both its treatment and prophylactic potential for the whole manic-depressive syndrome. In 1952, Delay and Deniker discovered the antipsychotic effects of chlorpromazine. Then, in 1956 and 1957, iproniazid, a monoamine oxidase inhibitor (MAOI), was shown to have antidepressant properties, and in 1958 Kuhn established the efficacy of the first tricyclic antidepressant, imipramine.

In subsequent years other antipsychotic, antiobsessive, and antidepressant medications have been developed. Even at this early stage of development, however, the antipsychotics and antidepressants have done nothing less than drastically reduce the population of mental patients throughout the whole world. Less dramatically but more importantly, they have greatly increased the population of ambulatory, socially functioning patients who have avoided hospitalization or protracted outpatient treatment.

In the early 1960s, William Sargant in the United Kingdom and Donald Klein in the United States launched a development that has added enormously to the revolutionary impact of the discovery of the modern psychotropic drugs. They established the usefulness of antidepressants in the treatment of certain neuroses and personality disorders, particularly in patients with phobic anxiety, hysterical, and anxious-depressive symptoms.[9] The demonstrated efficacy of the tricyclic and MAOI antidepressants with these classical neurotic symptoms ran counter to the then-prevailing notion that neurosis was a psychological, not a biological, phenomenon and therefore appropriately treated only with psychological interventions.

The recognition that neurotic and characterologic symptoms are no less responsive to drugs than psychotic symptoms has paved the way for a radical medicalization of all mental disorders. This is reflected in our current diagnostic nomenclature, DSM-III-R, which is a biologically rather than a psychodynamically based nosology. The trend has culminated in locating many of the personality disorders on the spectra of manic-depressive and schizophrenic illnesses and of defining the major anxiety neuroses, particularly agoraphobia and panic attacks, as variants of affective illness.[10] I shall discuss these topics more fully in Chapters 6 and 7.

Genetic studies, performed primarily in the Scandinavian countries during the 1950s through the 1970s, have powerfully strengthened the argument for a biological component in the etiology of the neuroses as well as the psychoses.[11] These studies have conclusively established that schizophrenic and manic-depressive illnesses are separable disorders, have telltale patterns of family inheritance, and have subpsychotic forms (e.g., schizotypal and borderline personality disorders) that fall on the schizophrenic or manic-depressive spectrum of disorders. These subpsychotic or neurotic variants—milder degrees of disturbances in mood and thought—are the symptom pictures that the children and other close relatives of psychotic patients often manifest at psychiatric evaluation, a fact that has significant clinical implications.

The tenets of the biomedical tradition are implicit in this brief review of its history. To summarize, neuroses and psychoses, from this perspective, are regarded at least in part as medical illnesses. This means that they are in significant measure the products of abnormalities in neurochemistry and neurophysiology. Treatment, therefore, involves the administration of physical and chemical agents that normalize these physiological processes. To be able to do this, the disorder must be correctly diagnosed in the medical sense, that is, given a label with specific connotations about symptom picture, etiology, course, and optimal treatment. Much more than in the learning theory and existential traditions, diagnostic labels are of vital importance in the biomedical tradition.

Hereditary factors are similarly important. Although many psychiatric symptoms are no doubt the result of toxic environmental events affecting brain and mind, the major syndromes and their neurotic variants represent chemical abnormalities that are propagated in families through genetic transmission. To medical doctors, therefore, a case of schizophrenia or manic-depressive disorder, no less than a case of diabetes, provides the occasion for family case-finding and genetic counseling. Biological psychiatrists are constantly on the lookout for mental disturbance in the siblings, parents, and children of depressed or schizophrenic patients. For example, when treating a manic-depressive adolescent girl, they often find a reclusive older brother who studies day and night and has no friends. Started on lithium or antidepressants, he miraculously begins to spend more time away from his studies in order to socialize with peers.

The case of Amanda, discussed in the last section, offers a further illustration of this approach. Because her father had been hospitalized for a "nervous breakdown," inquiries were made about his symptoms and diagnosis. It was determined that he manifested a combination of manic-depressive and schizophrenic features and thus had a schizoaffective disorder, which had responded to neuroleptic and lithium medication. Because Amanda manifested mood swings and disorganized, paranoid thinking, these symptoms were also regarded, in light of her father's illness, as possible borderline manifestations of an inherited schizoaffective disorder and consequently as good candidates for similar biological treatment. Fortunately, her symptoms of mood instability responded well to antidepressant and lithium medication, and her cognitive difficulties diminished on low doses of trifluoperazine. It is doubtful that the psychodynamic and existential interventions previously described would have been so successful in Amanda's case without concurrent psychoactive drug treatment. As the reader will see, learning theory and social interventions were also crucial to the outcome.

THE LEARNING THEORY SCHOOL

The learning theory school of mental treatment traces its origins to the early part of the twentieth century and the conditioning studies of Pavlov and Bekhterev. Among the major contributors to this approach have been Watson, Thorndike, Hull, Skinner, Tolman, Mowrer Kelly,

Wolpe, Bandura, and Beck.[12] The approach includes two major types of treatment: behavior therapy and cognitive therapy. What they have in common is a belief that mental symptoms are largely the result of faulty learning. Thus, they are not illnesses in the medical sense but rather a collection of bad habits that usually serve to reduce anxiety and drive level but at the cost of maladaptation. Behavior therapists focus their attention on bad habits of behavior (e.g., phobic avoidance) and the reinforcements that support them, whereas cognitive therapists focus primarily on the bad habits of thought and expectation (e.g., the erroneous ideas of danger and shame, that maintain the phobic fears). For both, the bad habits are the result of maladaptive conditioning experiences, either of the classical (Pavlovian, sign learning) or operant (Skinnerian, solution learning) types. Treatment therefore involves deconditioning the maladaptive thinking and behaving and relearning more adaptive routines, often in the form of assertive social skills. Such skills are developed by active rehearsal and shaping techniques.

For example, in this approach, neurotic depression might be defined as the result of learned helplessness, to use Seligman's term,[13] and learned negative attitudes about self-worth. Treatment, therefore, would involve overcoming the passive attitudes of feeling helpless and thinking negatively and replacing them with active, positive coping strategies. This might be accomplished by progressively cutting down on passive behaviors like excessive eating and drinking and practicing active ones like making previously unspoken demands on friends and colleagues and undertaking a vigorous exercise program. Such an approach places a premium on facing one's fears and practicing adaptive actions. Practice and homework are all important, and it is within the therapist's role to prod and guide the patient toward these accomplishments.

For example, in the treatment of Amanda, I gave numerous homework assignments to help her overcome her many symptoms of depression and disorganization. Because her grooming and homemaking were disaster areas of her life, she agreed to do her hair regularly, go on a proper diet, buy nicer clothes, and set up a schedule of regular housecleaning and laundering. She was given very bad marks for saying and thinking bad things about herself. She had to force herself to call up people to make social arrangements, and to take issue with her fiancé and boss whenever they made hurtful remarks to her. Because she sometimes overdid it, she had to learn to moderate some of these assertive behaviors.

This approach stands in sharp contrast to the psychodynamic tradition in which, for example, depression is regarded as the result of a regression to the oral phase of psychosexual development, precipitated by a loss and culminating in a state of ego depletion and anger directed toward parts of the self. Psychodynamic treatment of depression involves carrying through the normal grieving process by gaining awareness of the misdirected anger so that it can be suitably redirected to its real target and so that the mental energy mobilized can be used to repair the loss. In the process, the regression in psychosexual development is overcome.

Note that the processes referred to in the psychodynamic approach, both as to the genesis of symptoms and their treatment, mostly take place in the subjective realm of attitudes, feelings, and motives. In the learning theory tradition, by contrast, symptom formation and treatment goals all tend to be described in external behavioral terms, thereby making therapy less privately subjective and more amenable to controlled empirical observation.

Finally, it must be noted that cognitive and behavior therapy are activist. They require the patient to practice, to go out and face feared situations, to curb maladaptive behaviors, and to practice desired skills. Patients in this kind of therapy have homework assignments, just as in any educational venture. Because therapy here is education, the therapist is a teacher who gives the assignments and grades the homework. He or she prods the students to do the work and improve the performance. The therapist is highly directive and prescriptive.

In both the biomedical and psychodynamic traditions, in sharp contrast, treatment falls within the healing arts and sciences, not education and training. Particularly in the psychodynamic approach, the active direction involved in giving assignments is specifically forbidden as a damaging contaminant of the patient's autonomy and the therapeutic transference relationship. In taking issue with the psychodynamic viewpoint, however, the learning theorist would point out that the therapist is constantly and unavoidably contaminating the transference by his or her body language and other nonverbal behavior. Furthermore, the need for autonomy does not come into play until the individual has experienced sufficient dependency and direction, which many patients never have. Only with adequate parental direction does the patient or child develop the basis for self-direction.

THE SOCIAL SYSTEM SCHOOL

As made evident by Jerome Frank's definition of psychotherapy, reviewed in the last chapter, the presence of a group of fellow sufferers or witnesses has long been characteristic of mental healing rituals, particularly in their shamanistic and faith-healing forms. Even Charcot hypnotized away the hysterical symptoms of his patients at the Salpetrière in front of a large audience of awe-struck observers, and Semrad conducted his dramatic feats of "psychosurgery" in a public forum. Moreover, in Asian countries, even psychiatric hospitalization is a social event, almost always involving the simultaneous admission of family members to assist in the patient's care.

But this venerable social emphasis in psychotherapy experienced a decline in prestige with the advent of psychoanalysis and the dynamic tradition. In its thrust toward helping individuals become disembedded from the social matrix and thereby develop an individualized, reflective consciousness, the family and friendship networks were vigorously excluded from the process of analytic therapy. Therapists of this school would not even accept phone calls from the family or friends of patients, much less agree to see them together in the office. Psychodynamic therapy came to be thought of exclusively as *individual* psychotherapy.

Over the past 30 years or so, however, the social emphasis in psychotherapy has been recaptured, particularly in the family, group, and milieu therapy movements, the three main components of the social system tradition. Why this has occurred is only partially understood. Surely the breakdown of the family and the neighborhood and the disappearance of virtually all intermediate social structures from an increasingly fragmented society have played important roles in the emergence of resocializing forms of therapy. Already in the early part of this century, social approaches to psychotherapy were being envisioned. From a Marxist viewpoint, Adler began to think of pathogenesis and treatment as taking place in a social context. Moreno had started his experiments in psychodrama and group therapy by 1910 in Vienna and brought them to this country in 1925. And the American internist Joseph Pratt began didactic educational-support groups for tuberculosis patients by 1905.[14]

In contrast, the family therapy movement has been almost entirely a post–World War II phenomenon. It is noteworthy that many of the pioneers of this development—in particular, Ackerman, Bowen, Whitaker, and Minuchin[15]—were psychoanalytically trained and would no doubt regard their work with families to be post-Freudian, that is, utilizing and transcending rather than repudiating Freudian insights. Much the same could be said of Maxwell Jones, Stanton and Schwartz, John and Elaine Cumming, and other pioneers of milieu therapy.[16]

What the social approaches have in common is, first, the belief that because most psychopathology has been generated in a social context, a group or family setting is best suited to reevoking it for subsequent repair. But even when the pathology has been generated in a private context, the therapy group is likely to be unusually evocative because of the broad range of represented personalities, at least some of whom remind the patient of significant others from his or her past. When the key pathology derives from disturbances in early family structure, the family or group meeting can serve to recapitulate the original pathogenic circumstances with even greater force.

For example, a middle-aged woman who had been in individual therapy with me for some time also joined a group and immediately became explosively angry toward another woman and paranoid toward me for letting her "get away with murder." Almost instantly, the group has become her childhood family, the other woman her rejecting stepmother, and I her ineffectual father who failed to protect her from this "wicked witch." No prior description of her feelings toward her father and stepmother had prepared me for the intensity of her outburst. Similarly, Amanda, who was seen concurrently in group and individual therapy, repeatedly relived early pathogenic family experiences in the group setting. She often felt harshly criticized by members in terms reminiscent of her father's old behavior toward her. Corrective feedback from the group enabled her to get beyond these distortions.

The second tenet of the social system approach is that there are unique properties of family and group systems that are ideal for carrying out the treatment project. Among them is the propensity for groups to generate contagious affect, particularly of hope, support, and belief, all of which serve to strengthen the flagging will to health of the individual sufferer.[16] And the morale building the patient derives from simple group acceptance and the discovery that others have similar vulnerabilities cannot be overemphasized. Finally, the social system approach has unique advantages for carrying out certain kinds of interpersonal learning, for example, giving and receiving feedback and emotional support, taking leadership and followership roles, speaking to the point, and listening attentively. In all these tasks, family and group therapy provide effective contexts for doing the work: for the modeling, imitating, and shaping that learning theorists and, in different terms, psychodynamicists advocate so strongly.

What is unique about the social system approach, however, is its specifically social definition of pathology. So far I have discussed its advantages from the standpoint of doing therapy on the individual in the context of the family or group. But in its essence, the social school redefines the meaning of illness. According to it, mental illness is a property of the group or family as a whole, not of its individual members. The distress of individuals is mainly a reflection of system pathology.[18]

Thus, individuals are merely the symptom bearers of scapegoats for the larger group, whose leaders project their conflicts and systemic pathologies onto the vulnerable, caring members, whose main problem is their susceptibility to taking on the problems of others.

If this is so, then therapy is fundamentally an exercise in social reform. Obviously, such a notion applies best to families or naturally occurring groups, that is, those whose members live or work together in the extra-therapy world. In these naturalistic groupings, holograms and holographic interventions, which I will discuss in Chapter 5, apply with great effect.[19] According to these notions, not only does the pathology of the individual represent a microcosm of whole group pathology, but in special circumstances realizable by skillful therapists, repairing the pathology of the system repairs that of individuals, and vice versa.

The sick family or group is one in which the parents or leaders do not exercise their authority fairly or consistently, and in which the members do not have clear and appropriate role definitions and personal boundaries. Consequently, the emotional attachment of individual members to the group or family is either too close or too distant, so that it is difficult to belong and still have an adequate degree of both autonomy and support.

Repair of this social pathology requires the services of a social reformer who has the conceptual skills to redefine appropriate roles and boundaries, and the leadership qualities to get members to reorganize their group behavior and to stop imposing and receiving each other's projections.

SUMMARY

We have reviewed the significant tenets of the five main schools of mental treatment. We have seen that in the biomedical tradition, psychopathology is the result of medical disease, of biochemical and physiological abnormalities of brain function. Treatment, therefore, involves making a diagnosis of the disease and offering the physiological correctives, such as psychoactive medications. The therapist is a medical doctor, a practitioner of the science of medicine, an exemplar of Western scientific technique applied to the task of healing the human body and its most complex organ, the brain.

In the psychodynamic approach, pathology is the result of arrested psychological development and therefore the expression of immaturity. The arrest is brought on by the anxiety of conflict between different parts of the personality, with the result that one or more of these vital parts becomes split off from consciousness. Treatment is the gaining of insight into the unconscious contents and the conflict-anxiety responsible for their dissociation or repression. It is retrospectively analytic. The therapist is an objective understander and giver of insights into the patient's pathology.

In the learning theory tradition, pathology is the acquisition of maladaptive patterns of thinking and behaving as a result of faulty conditioning experiences. These learned bad habits often serve to reduce the pain of anxiety and frustrated drives but at the cost of maladaptation. Therapy is a process of deconditioning the bad habits and shaping new, more adaptive ones. This requires the patient to practice and curb certain behaviors, and to expose himself or herself repeatedly to feared situations. Because the paradigm is an educational one, the therapist is a directive teacher who gives homework assignments, and the patient is a receptive but active student who expects to be graded on his or her work.

In the social system approach, pathology is a property not of individuals, but of the encompassing social system. It is a reflection of abnormalities in leadership and role definition and in the quality of the boundaries, emotional attachments, and projection-introjection processes between members. Therapy is a restructuring of the dysfunctional social system, as a result of which the individual members experience positive benefits in social performance and contentment. The therapist in this tradition is a group leader, a social change agent, or a political reformer. As such, his or her mode of operation contrasts sharply with that of the therapist as doctor, insight giver, or teacher.

Finally, from the existential viewpoint, pathology is both the suffering of blocked creativity and a protective strategy for preserving the capacity to create in the future. The aim of existential therapy is to unblock the creative will by helping sufferers gain access to the true self in the deep unconscious and by developing a belief system that unleashes it. With the guidance of a mentor who has made progress in achieving this goal in his or her own life, existential sufferers are helped to understand the ultimate meaning of their existence and to find appropriate lifeworks, in the pursuit of which they realize their full creative potential.

The main points of this discussion are summarized in Table 1, where each of the schools or traditions is characterized in terms of healer role and the nature of pathology and treatment.

INTEGRATION

My position has been that each of these five traditions has made a major contribution to our understanding of mental illness and its treat-

Table 1. The Five Schools of Mental Treatment

School	Healer	Pathology	Treatment
Psychodynamic	Interpreter	Immaturity	Insight
Existential	Mentor	Blocked will	Self-realization
Biomedical	Physician	Illness	Medicine
Learning	Teacher	Bad habits	Relearning
Social system	Reformer	Group dysfunction	Restructure

ment. Each casts light on certain aspects of emotional distress and personal maladaptation and how they can be modified. The fact that they can be laid out in a table, with such a clear sense of getting at fundamental but different aspects of pathology, treatment, and the healer role, is already a step toward synthesizing the rival traditions into a unified approach. It is readily apparent that there is no irreconcilable conflict or redundancy among them. Like the contrasting wave and particle conceptions of light in quantum physics, they are all relevant, complementary accounts of the genesis of mental disorder, which always involves both bad chemistry and bad faith, both bad habits and bad social conditions.

But because the development of mental illness is multidimensional, so must its treatment be. Mental disorder has to be assailed in each of its hydralike forms, with the methods appropriate to each. It is only the order of the interventions that remains to be determined. What often happens is that the therapist first tries the modality that was most emphasized in his or her past training, and only if it fails to give satisfactory results are other approaches brought into play. What is needed instead is a rational scheme for sequencing treatment. Despite the fact that human beings and their situations are too complex and unpredictable to make strict adherence to any scheme practical, formulating an ideal sequence serves important purposes, not the least of which is to lower the chances of overlooking important etiological and treatment possibilities.

A further ordering of the five traditions provides a solution to the problem. If we range the five traditions on a continuum of concrete to abstract, basic to meaningful, molecular to molar, and objectively verifiable to subjectively individualized—in other words, on a continuum from biological to existential—we come up with the following hierarchy:

1. The biomedical approach
2. The learning theory approach
3. The psychodynamic approach

4. The social system approach
5. The existential approach

The five-part hierarchy determines a natural sequence of both understanding and treatment. The concrete to abstract, medical to metaphysical ordering is the most logical and common sequence in clinical practice. Because they address the most basic foundation of life, biomedical interventions come first; they typically precede the more complex and personal stages of treatment because they are often prerequisites to the effective utilization of the latter. The healer must first tend to physical lesions and chemical imbalances before dealing with the psychological traumas and spiritual disillusionments that accompany them.

The learning theory approach, with its emphasis on a training technology that, like medicine, safeguards all biological organisms—mice no less than men—naturally takes the second position in this healing chain. It helps ensure that the patient's more urgent survival needs are met by overcoming self-destructive habits and replacing them with adaptive skills. The central level, the psychodynamic approach, is the entry level into the unique problems of individual human minds, those centering on self-awareness and self-control. Once survival is assured, psychodynamic therapy improves the quality of life by promoting the maturation and integration of the individual.

But achieving mature, integrated individuality does not guarantee either social connection or existential meaning. Social membership is the province of the group, family, and milieu therapies, all of which organize the social matrix so that healthy love and work relationships are promoted. Finally, giving these love and work relationships higher meaning is the goal of existential therapy, the final integrator of all the other therapies. It seeks to harness all basic motives to the achievement of higher ideals, and it proceeds beyond a personal psychology to a suprapersonal belief system that unlocks the creative will. Existential therapy helps the individual find the kind of intimacy that promotes a unitive consciousness and the kind of lifework that, by expressing the universal self, makes a lasting contribution to the whole.

Thus, the approach I am advocating here, which I call bio-existential therapy, is serially pluralistic, as I have spelled out in other publications.[20] This integrative therapy looks at all patients serially from the biomedical, learning, psychodynamic, social, and existential levels, and it treats them in an orderly fashion by drawing on the resources of each level for the ultimate purpose of achieving the creativity of intimate connections, both to individuals and to larger wholes. Spelling out the parameters of bio-existential pluralism and showing how they further the ideals of all growth-seeking human beings are main goals of the book.

As already mentioned, what the reader will see in the next chapter, as I discuss the case of Beth and Howard, is that there are psychological impediments to following the logical sequence of the bio-existential approach. Human beings—at one and the same time biological, psychological, and existential creatures—cannot be fitted into rigid sequences or categories. As unique individuals with special requirements and needs, they must be taken at their own pace to realize their ideals.

NOTES

1. R. A. Harper, *The New Psychotherapies*, Englewood Cliffs, NJ: Prentice-Hall, 1975; C. H. Patterson, *Theories of Counseling and Psychotherapy*, 4th ed., New York: Harper and Row, 1986.
2. T. S. Kuhn, *The Structure of Scientific Revolutions*, 2nd ed., Chicago: University of Chicago Press, 1970.
3. Paul Starr, *The Social Transformation of American Medicine*, New York: Basic Books, 1982. See particularly Chapter 3, "The Consolidation of Professional Authority, 1850–1930, pp. 79–144.
4. E. M. Abroms, "Beyond Eclecticism," *Am. J. Psychiatry 140*:740–745, 1983. My first formulation of this position can be found in E. M. Abroms, "Psychiatric Serialism," *Compr. Psychiatry* 22:372–378, 1981.
5. R. May, E. Angel, H. F. Ellenberger, eds., *Existence: A New Dimension in Psychiatry and Psychology*, New York: Basic Books, 1958. I. D. Yalom, *Existential Psychotherapy*, New York: Basic Books, 1980.
6. A. F. Maslow, *Toward a Psychology of Being*, 2nd ed., Princeton, NJ: Van Nostrand, 1968; C. R. Rogers, *On Becoming a Person*, Boston: Houghton Mifflin, 1961.
7. G. Zilboorg, *A History of Medical Psychology*, New York: Norton, 1941; G. Mora, "Historical and Theoretical Trends in Psychiatry," in: H. I. Kaplan, A. M. Freedman, B. J. Sadock, *Comprehensive Textbook of Psychiatry*, 3rd ed., Baltimore: Williams and Wilkins, 1980.
8. See the introductory sections of Chapter 31 of *Comprehensive Textbook of Psychiatry*, op. cit., for a brief history of psychopharmacology.
9. W. Sargant, "The Treatment of Anxiety States and Atypical Depressions by the Monoamine Oxidase Inhibitor Drugs," *J. Neuropsychiatry* 3(Suppl. 1):96–103, 1962; D. F. Klein, "Delineation of Two Drug Responsive Anxiety Syndromes," *Psychopharmacologia 5*:397–508, 1964.
10. L. L. Heston, "The Genetics of Schizophrenia and Schizoid Disease," *Science 167*:249–256, 1970; H. S. Akiskal, "Subaffective Disorders: Dysthymic, Cyclothymic and Bipolar I Disorders in the 'Borderline' Realm," *Psychiatric Clin North America 4*:25–46, 1981.
11. S. S. Kety et al., "The Biological and Adoptive Families of Adopted Individuals Who Became Schizophrenic: Prevalence of Mental Illness and Other Characteristics," in L. C. Wynne et al., eds., *The Nature of Schizophrenia*, New York: John Wiley, 1978; I. I. Gottesman, "Schizophrenia and Genetics: Who Are We? Are You Sure?" in L. C. Wynne et al., eds., op. cit.; and J. Mendelwicz and J. D. Rainer, "Adoption Study

Supporting Genetic Transmission in Manic-Depressive Illness," *Nature 268*:327–329, 1977; R. J. Cadoret and G. Winokur, "Genetic Studies of Affective Disorders," in S. C. Draghi, F. F. Flach, eds., *The Nature and Treatment of Depression*, New York: John Wiley, 1975.

12. S. L. Garfield and A. E. Bergin, *Handbook of Psychotherapy and Behavior Change*, 2nd ed., parts III and IV, New York: John Wiley, 1978.
13. M. E. P. Seligman, *Helplessness: On Depression, Development, and Death*, San Francisco: W. H. Freeman, 1975.
14. I. D. Yalom, *The Theory and Practice of Group Psychotherapy*, 2nd ed., New York: Basic Books, 1975.
15. S. Minuchin, *Families and Family Therapy*, Cambridge, MA: Harvard University Press, 1974; A. Gurman and D. Kniskern, eds., *Handbook of Family Therapy*, New York: Brunner/Mazel, 1981.
16. G. M. Abroms, "Defining Milieu Therapy," *Arch Gen Psychiatry 21*:553–560, 1969.
17. See Yalom in note 13 above, especially the first four chapters.
18. This is an assumption common to virtually all systems of family therapy. The various systems are summarized by R. Simon, "Family Therapy," in H. I. Kaplan and B. J. Sadock, eds., *Comprehensive Textbook of Psychiatry*, 4th ed., Baltimore: Williams and Wilkins, 1985, pp. 1427–1432.
19. The idea of holograms derives from advanced physics and mathematics. It has been applied by Karl Pribram in his neurobiological studies of memory. For a study of the philosophical and psychological implications of this work, see K. H. Pribram, "The Neurobiologic Paradigm," in C. Eisdorfer et al., eds., *Models for Clinical Psychopathology*, New York: Spectrum Publications, 1981.
20. Abroms, op. cit., note 4 above.

CHAPTER 4

The Case of Beth and Howard

To paraphrase Tolstoy, happy relationships are all alike; every unhappy relationship is unhappy in its own way.[1] This is surely an oversimplification, but it gets at an important truth: Successful relationships have a large common ground, while failed ones are uniquely different, often coming undone because of a single flaw. All good love relationships are characterized by consistent mutual respect and affection; sharing of intimate feelings, interests, and fundamental values; and a strong commitment on both sides to preserve the bond. A deficiency or lack of reciprocity in any one of these attributes can doom an otherwise promising marriage. As we saw in Larry's case, recounted in Chapter 1, his second marriage was wrecked by disparate values, his first by an avoidant response to emotional closeness.

But Larry was able to achieve the outward structure of a bond, and he had two marriages to prove it. What he could not do was make the structure sound enough to endure. Because he could get married, however, the reparative processes of the standard psychiatric treatments—individual, group, couples, behavioral, and drug therapies—were sufficient to take him through the steps toward lasting intimacy.

The case I shall present in this chapter illustrates a much more serious relationship problem. Neither Beth nor Howard were able to sustain an intimate connection long enough to achieve a marital structure. All their relationships came apart before this milestone was reached, even though they both desperately wanted to get married and settle down. They were already into their 30s without even coming close, and both knew that a lonely fate lay in store for them unless fundamental changes were made. Although neither had grown up in a "psychotherapy culture," they were terrified enough of their dire prospects to take the plunge of seeking psychological help. Because of their instability in maintaining close ties—the hallmark of what are described as "borderline" conditions—an unusual approach was utilized on their behalf, a method I call outpatient milieu therapy.

MILIEU THERAPY

As a modern development of Pinel's moral treatment, originating in eighteenth-century France, milieu therapy was given its contemporary shape by Maxwell Jones in England, with further refinements introduced by Stanton and Schwartz and the Cummingses in the United States.[2] What all these behavioral scientists held in common was the idea that the successful psychotherapy of institutional patients requires that the focus of treatment be extended beyond individual therapy sessions into daily social behavior. As patients and staff work and socialize outside of formal sessions, their actions are brought under therapeutic observation and control. This is accomplished primarily by having community members report on each other at patient–staff group meetings. When sick behavior is observed, staff and fellow patients are shown how to give corrective feedback right at the time and place of occurrence. Obviously, such a 24-hour-a-day therapeutic community should be capable of generating a more intense and incisive therapeutic thrust than conventional treatment confined to 50-minute office visits, even of daily frequency.

This was my experience when some years ago I ran a general hospital psychiatric ward at the University of Wisconsin according to these principles.[3] In response to this highly intensive program, hospital patients often reorganized and returned to their normal lives with great alacrity. The key was broad democratic participation of the patients in their own treatment, thus making a virtue of the limited availability of doctors, nurses, and social workers. With staff help, the patients learned to present their own cases and the cases of their fellow patients at patient–staff meetings. They reported on each others' symptoms and were taught to do simple behavior therapy with each other, mutually discouraging sick and reinforcing healthy behaviors. The clarity and helpfulness of their reporting were taken as key indicators of therapeutic progress. To avoid the tone of "Big Brother is watching," great emphasis was placed on informed consent, avoidance of tattling, and heightened respect for privacy in matters that were nonessential to treatment.

Based on this experience, I have made two additions to the milieu therapy approach. First, I have shown that the therapeutic community, in the process of exemplifying a participatory value system, provides an ideal context for combining multiple treatment techniques to foster interactive social skills.[3] Its social therapy format makes it possible to synergize all available personnel and methods not only to combat symptoms but to model and develop satisfying personal relationships. The bane of a multidimensional treatment approach is the tendency for different therapists using different methods to work against each other. By enrolling all the participants in a common group therapy, however, the milieu approach fosters a harmony of goals, techniques, and relationships. Properly utilized, milieu therapy makes it possible for multiple therapists (who can include fellow patients) to combine modalities—psychodynamic, behavior, drug, group, and family therapy—in order to provide consistent, comprehensive treatment and, in the process, to teach the basic skills for sustaining intimacy.

Secondly, I have adapted the milieu approach to the outpatient setting. I have taken it out of the hospital and the institution and applied it to everyday social life. In a major abrogation of the traditional rules of outpatient therapy, which prohibit extra-therapy socializing and insist on individual privacy and confidentiality, members of the group are allowed, under supervision, to socialize outside of formal therapy sessions and then are required to report on each other's behavior at group meetings. To do this safely, the abrogated rules have been superseded by other rules, which, for example, set firm limits on sexual and financial dealings; I will discuss these more fully in Chapters 9 and 11. The most important of the new rules, however, is that all outside social get-togethers are to be regarded not as substitutes for "real" friendships, but as practice sessions for learning the relationship skills necessary to developing them. Even though these practice relationships cannot be prevented from becoming real, as the reader will soon see, such transformations are neither encouraged nor taken lightly.

Yet, no matter how carefully the rules are observed, the approach that I have used with patients like Beth and Howard entails serious risks of personal exploitation and cultishness. Consequently, it should not be undertaken without extensive training and supervision in group and milieu techniques and a heightened awareness of the dangers involved. With these considerations in mind, I offer the following case report, not to invite careless imitation, but as a cautious exploration of expanded treatment possibilities.

BETH

I first saw Beth at the end of July 1980. At first glance, I thought she was a model: She had a pretty face, a perfect figure, and stylish dress and grooming. She was 30 and never married but very popular with men. Her presenting complaint was that she was "drinking too much and becoming boisterous and telling lies." I subsequently found out that she was dating gangsters who frightened her by hiding guns in her apartment. But as I was painfully to discover over the next few years, Beth was often unable to describe her situation with clarity. I could not get a complete history and therefore initially missed the diagnosis. Because she had an obviously low mood and some disturbances of sleep and eating, I judged her to be depressed (dysthymic disorder, according to DSM-III[4]), took her drinking to be an attempt at self-medication, and started her on antidepressants. But she complained bitterly of side effects and very soon dropped out of treatment.

She reappeared 2 years later, looking about 10 years older. There were dark shadows under her eyes, and she was less carefully groomed. Her old complaints of excessive drinking and boisterousness were elaborated on. Bouts of drinking and overtalking tended to occur in episodes, preceded by a day or two of feeling tense and often accompanied by the onset of her menstrual period. During the episodes, she became angry, paranoid, and abusive toward her current boyfriend. She sometimes slapped him in the face and often was slapped back. Her thoughts raced, and she talked very fast, spitting out angry accusations. I realized at that point that she was not just an ordinary depressive but a manic-depressive.

In the past, her physical battling had been so intense that the police were summoned on several occasions. If she was not drinking, these episodes blew over in a day or two, but if she was, they could last a week. She desperately needed to get married, for she had been in and out of depression ever since her father had died a year and a half before. It was clear that she needed to replace him and have an intact family again, but her track record with men was terrible. All her romances had ended gruesomely.

Beth came from a close-knit, blue-collar Irish Catholic family and was the first of six children, now ranging in age from 32 to 19. Her father, a maintenance man, died at age 60 from kidney failure. His relationship with Beth was very warm and special; he often talked over family decisions with her instead of her mother. There was a strong history of alcoholism and depression in his family, which he himself proudly claimed to have avoided. At a family conference, her mother, age 62, appeared to be a very pleasant, self-effacing woman who had abdicated her authority in the family in favor of Beth.

What was most notable about Beth's mental status, besides her obvious mood swings, was a tendency to lose focus in her thinking: She rambled, became vague and disorganized, and occasionally had mildly delusional ideas of worthlessness or stupidity. But to counterbalance these weaknesses, she was uncannily intuitive, able to determine at a glance other peoples' strengths and intentions. Soon after entering a room full of people, she knew the main motivations of each person and what they really felt about one another, no matter what they pretended.

My corrected diagnosis in Beth's case was manic-depressive disorder with mixed borderline-schizotypal features.[4] My treatment plan was to integrate the interventions encompassed by the bio-existential approach: medications, cognitive-behavioral practice, psychodynamic understanding, social support, and the attainment of an adequate belief system.

My initial psychodynamic formulation began by noting that Beth had suffered a major developmental arrest in the capacity to have an intimate love relationship with a man. Her parents had been unable to set limits on her grandiose, out-of-control behavior. Moreover, she was in effect an "oedipal victor," still married to her father and forbidden to love anyone else. What she needed, prior to a love interest, was firm parental discipline.

Contributing to the picture of being out of control, her biological mood disorder made it difficult for her to tame her primitive sexual and aggressive drives, which were experienced and manifested by Beth as intense and animalistic. They too showed evidences of developmental arrest, for their expression was often immoderate and imprudent, manifested by difficulties in precision, focus, and logic. Also, in Piaget's terms, she had not fully reached the stage of formal operations, as she found it difficult to regard situations from multiple perspectives. Pulling all this information together, I thought that much of Beth's life was dominated by a primitive, angry, intimacy-destroying internal saboteur. Yet there were many unanswered questions about its origins. For instance, what was the early trauma and who were the identification figures that gave rise to this self-destructive part of her personality?

On the positive side, Beth had strong survival instincts and a great will to health and integrity. She was a fierce street fighter in battling against her self-destructive part. Considering her culturally and economically impoverished background, she showed great depth and strength of character to come for psychotherapy at all and then to open herself so fully to it. One might say that she had a powerful "watchful guardian," a split-off constructive subpersonality that was even stronger than her saboteur.

Course in Treatment

Started on lithium carbonate, Beth noted rapid quieting of the "raging" inside her and a cessation of all fighting with her lover, Bob. At the same time, however, she became profoundly dissatisfied with the immaturity of the relationship. She resolved to break up with him but found that she could not bring herself to do it. To support her in this decision, I started her in a therapy group, which had immediate payoffs.

First, the group gave her the encouragement and feedback to go out and get a better job. The members pointed out that her self-presentation was too tentative and vague to do well at interviews, and that she had to learn to defuse the competitive feelings that her beauty and sexuality aroused. Beth made the necessary corrections and soon had a more satisfactory work situation. The group was also firm about the self-destructiveness of her drinking and seeing Bob. Because her fellow therapy patients were obviously admirable people—they were successful, hardworking, and kind—she began to take pride in associating with them and to take their advice and feedback seriously. She began the process of identifying with and becoming part of the group will and thereby fortifying herself to combat the enemy within: her internal saboteur.

Soon drinking much less, Beth was encouraged to date someone besides Bob. Before long, she became involved with Tom and very quickly (like a runaway train) she was making plans to get married, even though Tom was not strong enough to be an appropriate partner. At the engagement party, she had a few drinks, and according to a fellow group member who was also present, she became cruelly grandiose and confronted Tom and her friends and relatives with all their faults. She told Tom that he was a "mama's boy" who was going to have trouble leaving home! Needless to say, Tom was shaken up by this penetrating attack on his masculine competence; when similar instances of Beth's arrogant sabotage surfaced over the next 2 weeks, he backed out of the relationship.

Beth was devastated. This was another failure in her love life and a terrible loss of face socially; now she was certain to be an old maid. She suffered a temporary regression in which she became grossly disorganized in her thinking and quasi-delusional about her "stupidity." These symptoms remitted with the addition of low-dose neuroleptic therapy to her regimen. Small doses of haloperidol (1–3 mg/day) made her feel much better able to cope with her trauma.

In the aftermath of the debacle, however, it came out that Beth's saboteur had done more than scare Tom off. It had also diverted her from taking her medications properly. Through some "misunderstanding," she had stopped her lithium altogether and lowered the dosage of her antidepressant. With prodding, she admitted that taking the lithium upset her stomach and made her feel defective, a topic I will discuss in Chapter 8. After an educational session on chemical imbalances, I explained that her breakup with Tom might not have occurred had she followed the prescribed regimen. Given the high stakes involved, she agreed to rededicate herself to taking her medication exactly at the dosages that we agreed upon and not listening to the dissenting voice of her saboteur.

Out of this defeat, Beth firmed up and began to show greater stability in her attitudes and behavior. She had paid heavily for her unreliability, a fact that she was helped to see clearly. From this time forward, she began to talk about getting well with great determination. She said she had found in me an adult who confronted her with the truth and held her to a high standard of behavior. Therefore, she could trust me to help her combat her primitive saboteur. This was a new kind of trust for Beth. Along with it came a growing sense of the importance of listening to sound advice and keeping her word. Even more important was her developing commitment to the value of psychological growth, which emerged as the guiding ideal of her life.

Following the broken engagement, her relationship with Howard, the other group member who was at the engagement party, took a significant turn. Because Howard was virtually a social recluse, Beth had offered some weeks back to introduce him to her social network and to fix him up with some of her girlfriends. He had tagged along to some of Beth's parties while she was dating Tom. After the breakup of the engagement, however, Howard took her out for dinner after a group meeting and told her how much he liked her and wanted to spend time alone with her.

Beth became "nauseous" at the prospect. She said, "I could never date a friend. Howard is like a buddy to me. It makes me sick to think that he is interested in me in that way." Close questioning revealed that she was afraid that if he got to know her intimately, he would find her worthless and discover that she used sex to gain power. In the process, the power of her internal saboteur became more evident: It dictated that only the needy, power-hungry part of her personality was allowed to become romantically involved, and then only with a derogated type of man. Her mature, caring part was not allowed to get close to anyone worthy of such feelings. I urged her to resist the saboteur's pressure to run away from Howard, and instead to overcome its sense of repulsion so that she could get to know him better. She greatly needed a supervised "practice" relationship to develop her capacity to sustain an intimate connection.

HOWARD

Howard was referred to me at the end of April 1982. He was a 35-year-old, never-married investment manager, already a senior partner in a growing firm. His chief complaint was that he had "trouble with women." He had gone through a string of relationships in which he withdrew at the point that a commitment was expected from him. Three weeks previously, he had done it again, causing great unhappiness to both himself and the woman in question. Worst of all, he found himself alone and socially reclusive once more. In sharp contrast to his social life, his professional life was going extremely well. It was perhaps too much of a good thing, for he was working 16 hours a day, 7 days a week.

He had two meaningful love affairs in his life. The first broke up when he returned from Vietnam to discover that she had fallen in love with someone else. The rejection made him depressed, which he managed by throwing himself into work. He dated his pattern of compulsive overwork from this time. Some years later, he began another serious relationship, which came unraveled when his girlfriend told him how much she loved him. In response, he found himself withdrawing emotionally and losing his feelings of affection. For the 3 years prior to entering therapy, he had reverted to having short-term relationships in which he was initially the pursuer, eliciting an affectionate response, and then the withdrawer.

Howard was the last of four children born to a second-generation German-American Protestant family. His father, now in his mid-70s, was a retired executive who treated his family as if they were rival members of a debating society. Howard constantly felt put down by him and the older brothers who took part in the debating game. His mother died in her early 50s (when he was 16) from cirrhosis of the liver and bleeding esophageal varices. Howard was uncertain about the role of alcoholism in her death, because her drinking problem was denied by the family. That she had been frequently incapacitated with rheumatoid arthritis and depression during his childhood, however, could not so easily be swept under the carpet. Two of Howard's siblings also had serious problems with drinking and depression.

Although Howard recalled his early years poorly, he did remember that he was often angrily defiant toward his mother, and at age 5, he started refusing to eat any of the food she offered him. His father had said he would eat when he got hungry enough, but this was a serious misjudgment. Howard went on a hunger strike and soon began to look emaciated. His parents capitulated and allowed him to feed himself whatever and whenever he wanted. Thus, from the age of 5 through 18, when he went into the service, he never again ate with the family, instead preparing for himself a severely restricted diet of peanut butter, french fries, and bacon, which he ate alone in the kitchen or his room. Even at the time of initial evaluation, he was still mildly anorectic. In contemplating the combination of illness and integrity involved in Howard's rebellious eating behavior, I considered the possibility that an individual's watchful guardian and internal saboteur might join forces. For by curtailing his eating, Howard not only developed a symptom but also a protection against swallowing the family's poisoned care.

At age 10 or 11, he was taken to a psychologist because of his eating problem and his tendency to hide for days at a time in a closet or attic. In fact, the police had been called in response to one of his disappearances. The psychologist's report alluded to his hatred of his mother, which he strongly denied when confronted. In fact, however, he could not bring himself to visit her on her deathbed, and after the funeral, he smashed up his room and had to be given an injection by the family doctor.

At age 15, Howard became involved with a delinquent gang that stripped cars and resold the parts. The next year his mother died, and in conjunction with his intense grief reaction, he moved out of the house into a motel, where he supported himself from the proceeds of the auto parts. He was never to live at home again, nor to attend regular high school. Shortly afterward, he got word from a family friend that the police were closing in on his gang and that he had better leave town. He immediately enlisted in the service and was sent to Vietnam. Other members of the gang stayed behind and went to jail.

This was to be the first of several occasions on which Howard's watchful guardian extricated him from great personal danger. In Vietnam, on two occasions he made fateful decisions to escape being killed by the Vietcong. When some fellow servicemen were going to beat him up for befriending a black soldier, he managed to get the military police to protect him without making specific charges—which surely would have gotten him killed, as one of the assailants later told him.

But the psychological impact of the Vietnam experience was profound. Howard realized that the world was a jungle from which the only escape was education and hard work. Inspired by his black friend, he began to read and think about the meaning of life. He enrolled in classes and quickly achieved his high school equivalency. After discharge he attended a local university, where he earned his bachelor's degree in business and then went on to get an MBA. He took a job with a small but growing investment firm, and by hard work and doing many favors for colleagues, he advanced rapidly and became a full partner by the time he came for treatment.

The psychiatric examination revealed an anxious, pale, immaculately dressed professional man who said of his mood: "I am extremely tense; I grind my teeth in my sleep and wake up exhausted." He had no other symptoms of depression or thought disturbance. His abstract thinking was permeated with personal concerns. For example, "A rolling stone gathers no moss" was interpreted to mean, "If you think of yourself alone, you won't end up with a family."

Although Howard clearly had significant character pathology I had difficulty fitting him into any of the DSM-III diagnostic categories. My hunch was that his early eating disturbance, phobic avoidance of people, and delinquent, truant behavior, as well as his later compulsive overwork, were all the outward masks of a well-defended, underlying biological depression. In favor of such a suspicion was the high incidence in his mother and siblings of depression and alcoholism, suggesting a genetic vulnerability in the family.

Equally important was the matter of the borderline dynamics of Howard's relationship difficulties. He harbored deep-seated resentment toward the deprivations of his childhood, which he managed by splitting off the hurt, angry part of himself from consciousness, the initial step in forming an internal saboteur. The rejection by his adolescent girlfriend reactivated this mechanism and led to two salient forms of acting out: compulsive overwork and passive-aggressive rejection of women. He went cold and turned away from women who offered to "feed" him love; thus, he extended his anorectic eating pathology into the realm of relationships. The reenactment of past deprivation at the time of a present offering of affection gave conclusive evidence of the workings of a split-off, love-rejecting subpersonality that subverted Howard's most deeply sought conscious aim of having a reciprocal love relationship.

Howard's assets were impressive. Basically a survivor, he was able to feed himself when others failed to do so. He exhibited the vital sense of timing always to escape extreme danger, evidence for the presence of a strong "watchful guardian." He identified with more adequate role models than his parents while in Vietnam and afterward displayed the intellectual and practical abilities, previously blocked, to get through college and graduate school to become a successful professional man.

The initial goal of treatment was to help Howard become capable of forming an enduring love relationship. To achieve that end I was prepared to utilize the entire bio-existential spectrum of therapies.

Course in Treatment

In the early months of our once-a-week meetings, Howard frequently canceled his appointments because of work pressures. Even though he knew the route to my office his saboteur would sometimes induce him to take a wrong turn, making him late for sessions. When he came he was often guarded and overly intellectual. In trying to resume his social life, he often sabotaged dates by showing up at the wrong time or place.

After surmounting these psycho-logistical problems, Howard went through a series of disastrous short-term relationships. He had a sure instinct for getting involved with depressed, alcoholic women. He once managed to pick up a woman at a ballgame who drank too much and had rheumatoid arthritis! He was impressed with the ingenuity he was demonstrating in finding women like his mother.

When we increased the frequency of his sessions to twice a week, he became more open about his feelings. He started to read more, and we began to exchange favorite books and records. But Howard often was unable to read the books or listen to the records that I gave him. My sense was that it was difficult for him to be "fed," even in this sublimated form. With notable exceptions, he always had to feed himself. Because he was socially isolated, I suggested that he join a therapy group with the hope that it might provide the warm, supportive family experience that he never received as a child. He also needed corrective feedback and peer pressure to stop overworking.

Initially, he was quite guarded and intellectual in the group, and he repeatedly questioned whether it had anything to offer him. These objections began to recede, however, once Beth joined. He looked her over with evident interest but considerable mistrust. Yet he jumped at Beth's suggestion that she include him in her social circle and fix him up with her girlfriends. On one of their early outings, Beth got drunk and became wildly manic, forgetting to look after Howard. He was furious and got in touch with some of the hurt feelings of neglect he had felt for his drunken mother as a child. He also shared his observations with the group about Beth's behavior, thus affording additional treatment opportunities for both of them. Although Howard was at first reluctant to have anything more to do with her, he was able to use the insight about the origins of his anger to make allowances for Beth and continue going to parties with her. He took on the job of reminding her not to drink and telling her when she was becoming too "boisterous." Thus, the treatment was beginning to go beyond the office walls out into the surrounding community.

After the breakup of Beth's engagement, he declared his romantic interest in her and evoked the feelings of repugnance that we have already mentioned. At my urging, she did agree, however reluctantly, not to run away from Howard, and he agreed to withstand her inevitable efforts to dump him.

BETH AND HOWARD

Beth had first taken Howard under her broad social wing approximately 6 months after they met each other in the group. Three months later came Howard's expression of interest in seeing her alone. The group encouraged Beth to go out with him, despite her disgust. With due warnings and an insistence on the platonic-practice and dutch-treat nature of their dating, I agreed to the arrangement. Because Howard was reclusive, he was given the responsibility for taking all the initiative in arranging the dates between them. He called repeatedly to make plans with Beth, but she put him off. It became very clear that getting them together, even for practice dates, was going to be like mating pandas!

In their respective individual sessions, I bolstered Howard against his feelings of rejection and Beth against her fears of not being in control of the relationship. It took a whole month before the first official date was consummated, despite the group's support and my constant maneuvering to help them get together. On the first date, Beth was mean and critical and very demanding, wanting doors opened and closed for her. When Howard reported her behavior, group members were sharply critical of Beth. It was clear that her high spirits intimidated Howard, who initially could not resist her finely honed talents for grabbing the upper hand. Once he learned to make demands and to give directions, however, Beth began to relax, and they had their first enjoyable, noncombative dates.

But Howard had to go into basic training to learn to become powerful enough to tame the wild saboteur in Beth. We began discussing the necessity of his prompt reaction to Beth's power grabbing, her need for limits, and his own insensitivity to being manipulated and difficulty in setting limits. We outlined strategies and tactics for accomplishing the task at hand.

Howard was sorely tested in the months ahead. On one date he unthinkingly went along with Beth's drinking. She then tried to lure him into bed, almost convincing him that the group's rule against sexual contact did not apply. Howard pulled back at the final moment, as he realized that giving in to her would jeopardize his relationships not only with me and the group but with Beth, who would have lost respect for him. On another occasion, Howard confided to Beth the shame he felt over getting involved in crime as a teenager, but instead of comforting him, Beth called him "a stupid jerk." I explained that Howard would not be able to trust her with his feelings again if she was not more supportive; besides, her behavior amounted to disowning her own shady past. As Beth became more responsive, Howard became more straightforward, and she in turn became more respectful.

Starting into the fifth month of their dating, they slipped into seeing each other more frequently than the group mandated. They found it harder and harder to be apart and not to touch each other. Howard confessed that he loved Beth and that he could barely control his sexual yearnings for her. Beth confessed that she loved him, too. She kept repeating, "He is such a nice person. He treats me so kindly. Nobody has ever treated me this way before." When this development was reported to the group, there was the expected range of reactions, from jealousy and resentment to admiration and vicarious happiness. But everyone agreed that this was no longer a practice relationship; either they would have to stop seeing each other, or one of them would have to leave the group. Not only was this the rule they had agreed to, but the intensity of their real romance was beginning to distract the group from its broader tasks.

After discussions and joint sessions, they finally decided that Beth would drop out, for Howard needed the group more than she did. She had a loving family and an extensive network of friends, while he had neither. The group hailed Beth's withdrawal as a step beyond narcissism and toward individuation.

Beth and Howard became physically intimate soon afterward and seriously began the process of becoming psychologically and spiritually intimate. The almost magical quality of their deepening love raised many questions. How did they develop such a strong attraction for each other, and why did I support their relationship against all the conventional rules of therapy? At first glance, they were too different to become a pair. But on closer inspection, it was apparent that they perfectly complemented each other, that they made good on each other's weaknesses. Beth was all instinct and intuition, areas of great deficit for Howard except in the realm of survival. She was constantly telling him "who was doing what to whom," vital information that he had previously lacked. And she was full of physical vitality and high spirits. Howard, on the other hand, was refined and retiring, a master of logical analysis and organized planning, major weaknesses in Beth's repertoire. Howard gave Beth the structure and culture she wanted and needed, and Beth gave Howard the intuitive understanding and vitality he lacked. And they both appreciated the gifts—no small thing.

As the old saying goes, "We are like the lame riding on the backs of the blind; we guide as they carry." But which one was lame and which blind? It changed from situation to situation. What really mattered was that they respected and were grateful to each other for the mutual help.

Forging the Bond

Nevertheless, forging an intimate bond between them was a stormy process. Threatened by Howard's growing influence in her life, Beth continually tried to subvert it by acting inconsiderately. For his part, Howard often became hastily impatient with Beth's cognitive problems. When he reported on her behavior, the group supported him in holding her more accountable but took issue with his abusive disdain, as corroborated by Beth's complaints to me. Thus, I was being provided with vital information about both of them, which I could utilize in their individual sessions to foster greater insight and maturity.

Most importantly, because of their membership in the treatment milieu, neither could disrupt their relationship with impunity. Both were caught in a web of connections and responsibilities. Their personal tie was embedded in a supportive social matrix. In the past, relationships had been held together by a network of social obligations, institutions, and customs. These had weakened sufficiently in modern times to make them ineffective factors in initiating and sustaining personal ties. The therapeutic milieu was now being used to provide the social glue that had been lost, to counteract the centrifugal forces that otherwise tend to pull relationships apart.

For therapy to fulfill this role adequately, however, Beth also needed the support of a group. After she left the original one she had continued to socialize with some of the members, but she needed more support and guidance than individuals could provide. This became painfully obvious after Beth and Howard became engaged and tried to make wedding plans. The bickering that flared up then became unmanageable; they agreed on a wedding date, but little else. Mainly because of Beth's combativeness, they fought bitterly about the arrangements: the location and type of ceremony, and whether or not family members were to be invited. Strongly provoked, Howard began to have second thoughts about marrying Beth. He wondered whether he really loved her or whether he had gotten caught up in the warm glow of support provided by the therapeutic milieu. Maybe he loved our sponsorship, but not Beth herself. Relieved that Howard was finally confronting this issue, which had always been lurking beneath the surface, I suggested they put off any wedding plans until they sorted out their feelings.

Beth was terribly disappointed but also aware that she had gotten out of control. Increased neuroleptic medication and individual therapy were inadequate to carry her through the crisis; she needed an effective surrogate family to stabilize her behavior. When this was explained, she readily agreed to go into one of my other groups. She promptly settled down and stopped battling with Howard. Her focus shifted to what it would take to pull off the marriage.

In the second group, she befriended Cheryl, a brilliant English professor at a local university, who dressed poorly and had no men in her life. Beth swooped her up, taking her clothes shopping and sending her to a good hairdresser. This effected a dramatic transformation of Cheryl's appearance. In return Cheryl validated Beth's intelligence and competence. Cheryl took Beth as her role model for being street-smart and feminine; Beth took Cheryl as her ideal of being book-smart. Basking in the glow of Cheryl's admiration, Beth dropped her guard and openly shared her insecurities about marrying a successful man. She made Cheryl her private consultant on all matters of social form and intellect. She also allowed Cheryl to keep me posted concerning obvious variations in her mood and thought disorders. In return, Beth reported on how Cheryl scared men away, which was apparent from their double dates. Thus, they became extremely valuable milieu resources for each other.

In the meanwhile, Howard had reconsidered his feelings and come to the realization that he loved Beth. Not only was he physically attracted to her, but they shared many interests and had great enjoyment together. Whatever the role of therapy in initiating their relationship, it now had a life of its own. He could not conceive of giving her up.

In the spring of 1986, Beth and Howard confided that they planned to get married in the coming week. Because Howard was too apprehensive to invite his family—"They will rain on my parade," he said—Beth agreed to a private ceremony in front of a justice of the peace. They asked if they could come by the office afterward. At the appointed time, they arrived to find most of the members of their groups, whom I had invited to share in the wedding cake and toasts. We all wished them a long and joyous life together. In effect, Beth and Howard received the blessings of their respective therapeutic "families."

Growth

Beth and Howard have been married for more than 5 years now, and they have two children. They have had many crises but have brought each one to a successful resolution. Over the years, their intimacy has grown deeper and fuller, particularly in their capacity to empathize with each other and to discuss their problems in managing their careers and raising the children.

Howard has gradually learned to pick up more quickly the signs of Beth's incipient hypomania and to help her rein in her behavior and structure her time. Beth's group played an invaluable role in the stabilization of her family life. For example, an older woman member helped her with the shopping and planning involved in furnishing and decorating the new house and, subsequently, with making preparations for having the first baby.

But the group played an even more fundamental role in Beth's growing self-confidence in the early years of the marriage. It gave her permission and support for living in a beautiful home, having a successful husband, and leading a comfortable life as wife and mother. Later it supported her in getting help so that she could go back to work. It combatted her poor self-image as a "dumb blonde, shanty Irish" who did not deserve to live well. Instead it gave her a place of honor by recognizing her rare intuitive talents and her great drive in making the most of her endowment. She blossomed in response to the milieu's nourishing but demanding support.

Predictably, Howard began to distance himself once he was safely married. He went through periods when he withdrew emotionally and became inattentive in social situations. Members from their respective groups who double-dated and partied with them reported that Howard often picked on Beth in public and that she would retaliate by complaining about his loud stereo and his late hours at the office. Now that he had found a home, the split-off resentful and unloved child in him became more manifest. Healing Howard's split was the final major challenge facing us. Fortunately, Beth, along with the milieu members, provided the necessary support.

Just as Howard had earlier reported on Beth's symptomatic behavior, now she reported on his. She noted that his partners treated him in a demeaning manner at social gatherings—more like a mascot than an equal—and that he did not fight back. Similarly, he was always seeking the approval of his father at family affairs, but when he did not get it, he became passive-aggressive (he pouted, showed up late and left early) rather than effectively assertive. He needed to stand up to his partners and his family, to demonstrate that he would not continue the relationships on these terms. With the encouragement of his group, he decided to break the pattern by temporarily cutting off from his family, refusing all invitations to get together until he could become independent of his father's approval. Howard wrote his father a respectful but firm letter explaining his need for a time-out in their relationship, and Beth fielded the outraged phone calls that resulted.

But carrying out this plan precipitated a clinical depression. Howard became dejected, slept poorly, and came down with a series of inflammations. Within a 3-week period, he suffered from streptococcal pharyngitis, a severe cold, and a tender joint. But when I tried to start him on the antidepressant nortriptyline to get him through this time, he became very suspicious, initially declining to follow my recommendation. When he finally decided to try it, he complained so strongly of its sedative effects that it had to be discontinued. Yet all psychological efforts to reverse his deepening depression failed. Insight into the nature of his losses was entirely ineffective, as were efforts to socialize with friends and to adhere to a vigorous exercise program. He lost interest in his work, ate poorly, and withdrew socially.

Now I was certain he had a biological depression requiring medication. He needed not only the pharmacological benefits of medication but also the psychological ones, for I knew intuitively that his resistance to taking psychoactive medicine was a hologram of his general resistance to being fed and nourished by intimates. Breaking through this barrier would effectively repair his core pathology. In other words, an effective course of antidepressants in Howard's case would serve as a "holographic intervention": it would address the whole bio-existential range of his disorder. But how was I to overcome his resistance?

Soon the opening presented itself. I was about to lend him another record, which he would typically fail to enjoy, when it occurred to me to give him two competing versions of the same symphony. As an expression of his personality split, he manifested splitting in his response, finding one of the discs all good and the other all bad. I knew then that the battle to feed him had been won. I immediately made him a present of the preferred disc, which he was too stunned to refuse. Soon afterward,

I convinced him to try the new antidepressant fluoxetine (Prozac) and to compare its effects with the hated nortriptyline. True to form, he appreciated the superiority of Prozac: it had fewer side effects and its positive effects, including antiobsessional properties, were particularly useful for him. With my coaxing he acquiesced in taking it regularly and allowing it to work.

The medication took effect with dramatic consequences. Paradoxically, as he now felt stronger and less depressed, he was able to tolerate getting in touch with how traumatically depressed he had been as a child. He relived the intolerable grief and rage caused by his parents' negligence, by his mother's inability to feed and care for him properly, and he remembered how this pain went numb as his hurt self was first split off from consciousness. He saw clearly that going on the hunger strike at age 5 was his reproachful demonstration that he could do a better job of feeding himself. Thus, toward the end of his therapy rather than at the beginning, Howard was induced to take in the healing psychobiological nourishment that he had missed out on as a child and that he had subsequently rejected in angry defiance.

As he assuaged the feelings of the hurt, depressed child in him, Howard's mature self gained access to its outraged demandingness and began to use it to get contemporary adults—his wife and partners—to "feed" him better. Making conscious the proper target of his old resentment, he stopped taking it out on Beth, and he became both increasingly affectionate and appropriately demanding toward her. At the same time he began diminishing his compulsive overwork. He started to take whole weekends off and to come home in time for dinner during the week, and he found time to have lunch with men from his or Beth's group.

In one of the most curious developments of this period, Beth's family began to treat him with ever greater deference and respect, just as he was breaking away from his own family and the "hurt, deprived little boy" role he had played in it. Beth's siblings symbolized their regard for Howard by insisting that he occupy the head place at all family dinners—in the very chair that their deceased father had once occupied! Thus, Beth had accomplished her mission of filling the void left by her dead father and making her family whole again; and Howard had replaced his old rejecting, intimidating family with a more loving one that accepted (and even insisted upon) his position of leadership.

Because he now needed his business partners less as a source of family love, he began to look at them more critically. He developed serious reservations about the quality of their work and their values. He, therefore, took steps to get into a leadership position so that he could improve the whole organization. In fighting the battles that ensued, he tapped into newly available stores of assertiveness to set limits and effect change, in the process becoming director of the firm. Subsequently he reconnected with his own family on very different, adult terms. He realized that his father was now an old man who had already given what he could and therefore should be honored as he was.

In the meanwhile Beth, once she was certain that she could manage her household, became restless to do something outside it. She had a natural gift for interior decoration; friends had always sought her help in decorating their homes and apartments. To professionalize her talents, however, she needed to get some formal training and to address the marketing and other business issues involved. Initially lacking the confidence for the undertaking, she derived great comfort from Howard's support and his offer to do her books for her once she got started. Meanwhile, Cheryl helped her write the requisite letters and applications. With their encouragement and the group's, Beth gradually got the business off the ground. The resulting boost in her self-assurance spilled over into her relationship with Howard, whose career success no longer intimidated her.

As their psychotherapy wound down, Beth and Howard began to form their own network of friends outside the therapeutic milieu and therefore to socialize less and less with fellow patients. Beth was particularly proud of her own group of young mothers, some of whom encouraged her and Howard to join their athletic club. Still on her lithium, she continues to see me periodically for routine medication checks. Although they have both finished their formal psychotherapy, Beth and Howard continue to work on their personal growth. She strives to become better organized, more responsive to her husband's and children's needs, and more competent in her work. Howard has set himself the task of becoming a better manager of people and his own time, a busy executive who increasingly has quality time with his wife and children.

What I shall try to do in the chapter ahead is to provide more of a theoretical basis for how the case of Beth and Howard was managed and why it proved so successful. In particular, I will examine the diagnostic and treatment staging issues and the abrogation of traditional therapy rules that were responsible for the efficacy of the pluralistic approach that I have illustrated here.

NOTES

1. The original quote from the opening of Tolstoy's *Anna Karenina* is "Happy families are all alike; every unhappy family is unhappy in its own way."

2. Maxwell Jones, *The Therapeutic Community*, New York: Basic Books, 1953; Alfred Stanton and Morris Schwartz, *The Mental Hospital*, New York: Basic Books, 1954; John Cumming and Elaine Cumming, *Ego and Milieu*, New York: Atherton, 1962.
3. See G. M. Abroms, "Defining Milieu Therapy," *Arch Gen Psychiat* 21:553–560, 1969; and G. M. Abroms and N. S. Greenfeld, *The New Hospital Psychiatry*, New York: Academic Press, 1971.
4. American Psychiatric Association, *Diagnostic and Statistical Manual of Mental Disorders*, 3rd ed., Washington, DC: APA, 1980.

CHAPTER 5

The History and the Hologram

The past is the best predictor of the future. This maxim is the guiding impetus behind the case history in psychotherapy. Evaluating the patient's current difficulties in light of his or her past history is the main function of the initial evaluation. What one typically discovers in these diagnostic sessions is that both the healthy and neurotic patterns of an individual's life are laid down very early and then relived over and over again. For example, in the last chapter, we saw that Howard, as early as age 5, began to feed himself and to extricate himself from life-threatening dangers. He also repeatedly distanced himself from needy women, starting with his alcoholic mother. I had to be mindful of these facts in order to design an effective treatment plan. Similarly, Larry, discussed in Chapter 1, recurrently experienced disruptive anger and depression every time he became involved in an intimate relationship. Yet he also manifested, from an early age, sound values and the capacity for sustained hard work.

Thus, what we discover from the client's case history is that characteristic patterns tend to recur, that individuals act out repetitive scenarios, both good and bad. To discover what these are before they play out again puts patient and therapist in a commanding position either to prevent an unwanted recurrence or to facilitate a desirable one that is about to happen. The result can be the creation of better scenarios for the future. Beyond symptom reduction this is the primary aim of a comprehensive psychotherapy: disrupting old, less adaptive behavior patterns and replacing them with new, more fulfilling ones.

To achieve this goal, the therapist must have the tools to see beyond the patient's presenting complaints to discover major underlying themes. Foremost among these tools is the ability to perform a careful psychiatric

Table 2. Outline of the Psychiatric Examination

1. Identifying Characteristics of Patient
2. Informants
3. Chief Complaint
4. Present Illness
5. Past History
   a. Growth and development
   b. Illness and health; drug history
   c. Education
   d. Career course
   e. Social relationships
   f. Sexual experience
   g. Legal entanglements
6. Family History
   a. Demographic data
   b. Quality and pattern of relationships
   c. Incidence of mental disorder
7. Mental Status Examination
   a. Appearance and behavior
   b. Form and content of thought
   c. Perceptual disturbances
   d. Affect and mood statement
   e. Cognitive-intellectual functions
8. Diagnosis
9. Etiological Formulation and Treatment Plan
10. Course in Treatment

history and mental status examination. The form of this study is outlined in Table 2 and discussed at great length in standard textbooks of psychiatry, which the reader is advised to consult.[1]

A review of Chapter 4 will reveal that this was the outline I roughly followed in presenting the cases of Beth and Howard. What I want to do in this chapter is to show how focusing on various aspects of this examination—particularly the patient's chief complaint, present illness, and family and past history—can elucidate the recurrent patterns the therapist needs to know in order to carry out effective treatment. In essence, these patterns are arrived at by utilizing two main hypotheses of interpretation: the theory of reenactment and the idea of the hologram. Examining the clinical phenomena in accordance with these two principles can tell us, sometimes with uncanny accuracy, what lies in store for the patient unless changes are made. Moreover, such an analysis can help us determine what changes might be effective.

THE THEORY OF REENACTMENT

A corollary of so-called object-relations theory,[2] the theory of reenactment—which hypothesizes that individuals will continually relive early formative relationships—has its origins in Freud's notion of the repetition compulsion, most clearly discussed in *Beyond the Pleasure Principle*.[3] Freud maintained that the conservative function of the instincts, which constantly seeks to restore and prolong everything that has existed in the past, can override their pleasure-seeking function and continue to bring back previously repressed painful experiences. This tendency is thus an essential prerequisite of effective psychodynamic treatment, for it ensures that in a properly managed psychotherapy, the crucial pathogenic experiences and relationships from childhood will be relived with the therapist and therapy exposed to corrective repairs.

But it is also the basis for the patterning of peoples' lives outside of therapy, giving the illusion that they are governed by an external fate. For example, Elena, a successful architect who had experienced the devastation of a yearlong incarceration in a remote contagious-disease hospital at age 7, subsequently was fired or angrily resigned (for reasons she was unaware of) from five different jobs as an adult, each time reexperiencing the same original sense of banishment. This phenomenon has achieved popular contemporary expression in the notion, already alluded to, that people have lifescripts or scenarios that they repeatedly live out.

The essential Freudian idea, however, is that these toward and untoward events, which constitute our fate, are not happening to us; we are in fact bringing them about. "We are actually ourselves bringing about what seems to be happening to us," as Thomas Mann articulated Schopenhauer's original "Freudian" insight.[4] But how do we accomplish such a feat? As far as untoward events are concerned, we succeed in part by being selectively attracted to individuals and situations that have the potential for harming us and then prodding them to do so—all unconsciously, of course. Thus, Larry in Chapter 1 picked employers and love partners with the potential for mistreating him, and then he provoked abusive behavior in them, on the model of his father's cruelty toward him in childhood.

The psychodynamic and learning theory accounts of projective identification, selective reinforcement, and behavioral shaping give operational significance to Freud's crucial insight, making sense of how we get others to do our unconscious bidding. By utilizing just such mechanisms, Freud himself may have shaped his destiny to be repeatedly "abandoned in anger after a time by each of his protégés" and betrayed with ingratitude by his friends.[5] This continually replayed script characterized his relationships with Breuer, Fliess, Adler, Jung, Rank, and several others. What Freud's contribution was in achieving this result is not available to us, but we can get answers from the patients who enter therapy with similar patterns and are able to trace them back to their origins.

The striking thing we discover about these reenactors is that they have often experienced early traumatic grief that was attenuated by dissociative splitting, the process most closely associated with the work of Janet and nineteenth-century French psychiatry, as was discussed in Chapter 2. One possible product of splitting is a "watchful guardian" subpersonality that unconsciously protects us from harm. More telling for pathology is the emergence of an angry, hurt, and vengeful internal saboteur that reenacts our characteristic self-defeating scenarios. This dissociated part keeps undermining the adult self's best-laid plans for success, or robs such success of enjoyment by inducing guilt and doubt about it. Thus, the destructive subpersonality imposes on the individual's life a harsh destiny. It continues to act out its hidden, subversive agenda until, through psychotherapy, it is coaxed into assuming a more constructive role in a unified personality.

A second, crucial aspect of reenactment is that the individual can play either role in reliving an early traumatic relationship. For example, among all his failed relationships, Larry was often the victim of abuse, just as he was in childhood with his father. But sometimes he was the perpetrator, enacting the role his father had originally played rather than his own. Thus, in reliving early relationships, one can identify with either the aggressor or the victim, depending on the contingencies of the situation. It is the relationship pattern, not a particular part in it, that is relived. Such a notion greatly expands our understanding of internal saboteurs and their patterns of reenactment. Saboteurs are not just angry reactors to mistreatment who are trying to redress a wrong. In some cases, they have also identified with the wrongdoer, taking on its hateful personality attributes—and thus sometimes doing unto others what was done to them, and sometimes getting the others to do it to them again.

Third, discerning a relationship pattern from the concrete data of a person's history is a high-order abstraction that is not always easy to achieve. The patient, caught up in the swirling currents of living his or her daily life, finds it virtually impossible to stand outside the action to see the plot structure. And the therapist may likewise be too caught up in the details of the case to separate figure from ground. A high level of attention and sensitivity to patterns is required. This can be developed by diligent practice in looking for them as patients tell their stories, by taking extensive case notes and constantly reviewing them, and by talking over cases with supervisors and colleagues, all in pursuit of ferreting out the guiding scenarios.

Even though the scenarios are typically located outside patients' awareness, they still cannot help revealing them to the attuned observer. Internal saboteurs are always dropping clues as to their hidden purposes. If therapists can learn to listen "with the third ear," they can discern these hidden agendas, and they can locate the portals that are open to therapeutic influence. Nothing is more helpful to this process than picking out the guiding *holograms* of the patient's life.

HOLOGRAMS AND HOLOGRAPHY

Derived from the philosophies of Leibniz and Whitehead and certain conceptions in quantum physics, holography was introduced to behavioral science by Karl Pribram, who first used it as a metaphor to explain the widely distributed nature of memory traces in the brain and the consequent resilience of past learning to focal brain damage.[6] Holographically distributed patterns are those in which each part (e.g., a piece of a photographic diffraction film or an isolated body cell) contains information about what is stored in all other parts, thus permitting one to reconstruct the whole photograph or the entire genetic code of the organism from each of its pieces. Thus, a hologram is a representation of an object or event in which every part contains sufficient information to characterize the whole. Each part represents the whole, and the whole implies each part.

As Pribram recognized, this is a promising metaphor for understanding certain aspects of behavior. Human beings are always saying and doing little things that show their "true colors," that represent their whole personality structure. For example, the distinguished captain of industry who tells a racist joke at a party may thereby provide a diagnostic biopsy of the dark, mean core of his character, subsequently observed in such other manifestations as the exploitative, condescending way he treats his employees. Similarly, the Freudian analysis of dreams and parapraxes is, in one sense, a search for certain kinds of holograms: those that represent the individual's whole system of unconscious drives and wishes. And creative psychotherapists like Robert Pottash, whose work I discussed in Chapter 2, typically scrutinize the details of patients' clinical histories for representative holograms of their overall motivation and ability to make positive changes.

In developing this prior work, I would offer the following theory: Asked to follow certain instructions, patients will reveal in their microbehaviors their unconscious macrointentions with respect to the course of psychotherapy. In other words, if patients are asked to perform certain therapeutic tasks, they cannot help revealing their total unconscious plan for treatment outcome—how they want it to turn out, and what interventions they will reject or respond to. Moreover, if therapists are properly attuned to reading these omens, they can either revise their expectations of treatment or take corrective actions to elevate the goals.

What are the tasks that induce patients to reveal these holograms? They are typically quite straightforward: calling for and agreeing to an appointment, following directions to reach the office, showing up and leaving on time, explaining why they have come for help, following treatment directions, and paying bills on time. In addition, as I will discuss in Chapter 9, we can increase the yield of holograms by bending some of the standard rules of therapy, for example, by getting patients to accept food, drink, and presents from us and then examining the evoked responses. Thus, as the reader saw in Chapter 4, Howard's initially negative response to offered recordings provided a key diagnostic and treatment hologram for overcoming his core anorectic pathology.

At this point, we need to run through several holograms to get a better feel for how they are read. As a first example, a new patient complained about how long it took to drive to my office. When she described her route, I pointed out that there was a much quicker way. After I described it, however, she said she preferred to stick to the old way that she knew. My sudden dread that this refusal was a hologram of her lack of openness to change in therapy was soon borne out by her general resistance to new ideas and approaches to solving her problems. Rather than new departures, therapy with her had to involve a shoring up and refinement of old defenses and coping methods. Similarly, despite carefully described, plainly marked signposts, a patient who had seen me once two years before simply could not find his way to my office. After two phone calls that still did not bring him to his destination, I decided to stand at the roadside to flag him down. He raced by two times before I finally got his attention. Of the possible cognitive and motivational bases for this difficulty, none gave promise of a serious ability to face his problems in therapy. In fact, he subsequently sent his wife and other family members to see me rather than go himself!

To take a contrasting example, Cheryl (Beth's depressed friend), urged by me to take action to improve her life, abruptly moved from her ramshackle apartment in a slum to a nice one in a good neighborhood, despite severe anxiety and self-doubts caused by the change. As

I hoped at the time, this action turned out to be a hologram of her therapeutic course: she subsequently made a series of painful upgrading moves that presaged major improvements in the quality of her life, not only in her mood but in her level of activity, standard of living, and love satisfaction. At the opposite end of the spectrum, a patient who was stuck in a refractory depression stopped her antidepressant medication because of minor symptoms of dry mouth, even though her mood had clearly improved on it. After providing this hologram, she went on to find something intolerably wrong with three subsequent medications and an easy physical conditioning program.

Thus, as psychotherapists, we are constantly on the lookout for holograms that give early warning of therapeutic outcome. At their best, such holograms capture the patient's qualities of initiative, motivation, cooperation, flexibility, and persistence in overcoming crises and achieving psychological growth. By watching how patients meet the basic expectations of therapy, such as showing up and following directions, we are given an early indication of their overall will to psychological health.

I have so far mainly looked at holograms for their prognostic significance: what is likely to happen in therapy if the patient's unconscious agenda is allowed to hold sway. But holograms can also tell us what interventions need to be made to change the prognosis. The fact that Howard went on a hunger strike at age 5 and subsequently fed himself tells us that he must learn to accept being fed in order to overcome his personality disorder. The holographic intervention I designed to achieve this result was to get him to accept gifts of records from me. This eventually led to his accepting antidepressant medication and finally to a deeper swallowing of Beth's love and nurturance.

What is important to realize is that to the attuned therapist, patients are always dropping hints, not only about their hidden intentions but also about their secret requirements for getting well. The unsuccessful attorney who bursts into my consulting room without knocking, despite clear instructions as to the location of my waiting room, needs a great deal of attention paid to proper procedures—what channels to go through, what sequence of steps to take—if therapy is to help him succeed in his profession. The patient who always pays her bills long before they are due, no less than the one who is always late, needs therapeutic attention—in the first instance to become less compulsive, in the second to become more so. The patient who "accidentally" takes the therapist's chair at the group meeting will have to be put in his or her place in several holographic ways. The patient who will never drink the therapist's coffee or tea, instead always bringing his own from the next-door coffee shop, or the one who gulps down the whole pot, will need, as Howard did, specific attention paid to his underlying anorectic or bulimic mechanisms.

In espousing these quick jumps to far-reaching conclusions, I must enter an obvious caveat: Attributing holographic significance to isolated events and small happenings is subject to significant error. As always when making large inferential leaps, the therapist must be constantly on the lookout for corroborative evidence and must be willing to abandon those theories that fail to generate supportive evidence and fruitful consequences. Yet, with this proviso, the existence of holograms is a great aid to the therapist's work. It holds out the possibility that human beings can show their true colors very quickly, and that the attuned therapist can take advantage of these revelations to adjust treatment goals and strategies. The individual who cannot bring herself to visit her dying friend or who shies away from her recently divorced colleague is a very different therapeutic prospect, and one in need of very special attention, from one who becomes readily and steadily available in such crises. In their everyday experiences of life, the ordinary happenings and stresses, human beings say and do things that serve as holograms of their basic personalities and intentions. To upgrade the quality of their work, therapists must become attentive to these holograms and extract their fullest prognostic and therapeutic implications.

Armed by the interpretive tools that the idea of the hologram and the theory of reenactment provide, we can now examine more fruitfully the format of the case study outline and see how the insights derived from these principles were used in managing the case of Beth and Howard.

THE CHIEF COMPLAINT

The presenting complaint, which is the patient's reason in his or her own words for coming to treatment, is perhaps the single most fruitful source of holograms available to the therapist. Often, in a very compressed phrase, the patient reveals the quality of his or her self-awareness and attitudes toward emotional distress, the need for help, and crucial figures in his or her life. Howard's chief complaint was, "I am having trouble with women." He did not say that he just broke up with someone and that he felt despondent about it or that he was having trouble maintaining a close relationship because he withdrew every time he elicited needy affection. The style of the complaint is quite distinct: "women" is impersonal, emotionally distanced, and disparaging in a highly generalized way; "trouble" is vague, unpsychological, and guarded. The picture that emerges is of an unpsychological, emotionally constricted young man who has poor self-awareness and ambivalent, aloof relationships with women, whom he regards as sources of trouble rather than as nourishing warmth. He is going to need a form of therapy that presents women in a richer, more enchanting light, and one that knows how to get around his lack of psychological insight. The fact that he is a successful professional man despite obvious arrests in emotional development is strong evidence that he possesses a high level of conflict-free talent for his chosen career.

Beth's chief complaint was, "I am drinking too much and then become boisterous and tell lies." She is out of control, wild, instinctual, alcoholic, and manic. Thus, while Howard is constricted and needs drawing out, Beth is expansive and needs reining in. This oddly phrased chief complaint from an Irish Catholic woman also has the flavor of the confessional about it, as in "Father, I have lied and been disrespectful to my parents." Somehow the therapist, if he is to succeed with her, had better summon up some added priestly authority—an adequate replacement for the church and the father she had earlier lost. Note also her choice of the word *boisterous;* it is boastful and pretentious. She is obviously proud of being wild and therefore will not give it up without great humiliation, which will have to be carefully assuaged.

Reading chief complaints in this way (i.e., for their holographic significance) is clearly an intuitive, artistic activity. Conclusions must be jumped to by association. They cannot initially be subjected to verification procedures. We are involved here in the logic of discovery, not the logic of proof, to use Karl Popper's distinction.[7] Learning to make these discoveries requires the kind of practice that can be achieved only by taking extensive notes of therapy cases and subsequently comparing the initial chief complaints with the long-range outcomes. The therapist is shocked to discover that quite often virtually everything about the clinical course was derivable from the initial statement. This sensitization procedure is one of the main ways that therapists learn to recognize the existence of holograms in the microcosmic utterances and actions of their patients.

For instance, a middle-aged man's presenting complaint was, "My wife says I'm depressed." He quietly dropped out of treatment a few weeks later unable to form a meaningful alliance with the therapist. In retrospect, the outcome was predictable, because the complaint reflected the patient's refusal or inability to take responsibility for his behavior and therefore for changing it. Either he did not know he was depressed and was dependent on his wife's judgment in the matter, or he did know but would not put himself on the line for making changes, reserving the right to take an oppositional stance toward the therapist. On the face of it, neither of these alternatives was a favorable omen for therapy.

Nevertheless, patients who present with unfavorable holograms may still be able to rise above them if they are given the right kind of help. For example, a women opened with, "My husband says I'm always down in the dumps, but I don't know what he's talking about; I felt fine." In fact, she looked morose, had low energy, poor sleep, and a pessimistic outlook. With reluctance, she accepted the diagnosis of depression and started taking antidepressant medication. On protriptyline (Vivactil) at 30 mg a day, she became animated and said she felt wonderful. "My God!" she said, "I must have been depressed for years and didn't know it."

Thus, a repeated word of caution about interpreting holograms: One must constantly check out and be prepared to revise the hasty conclusions drawn from such small samples of behavior. In employing the hypothetico-deductive method of science, we must be willing to entertain sequentially a multitude of theories, many of which will turn out to be wrong, rather than cautiously reserve judgment until incontrovertible evidence emerges. As John Locke taught us, truth proceeds more readily from error than uncertainty.

To take another example, a 47-year-old merchant presented with this startling question: "I'm thinking of leaving my wife, selling my business, and going to law school. Am I crazy?" I initially thought so. At the very least, it sounded rash, the sort of thing men say but later think better of when they are going through a midlife crisis. In favor of this interpretation was the fact that he had never even finished college. Five years later, however, he graduated at the top of his law class and went on to become a successful attorney. What had I missed? That he was a near genius who had shut down during adolescence when his father committed suicide, a Rip Van Winkle who was now awakening in midlife. With the help of a photographic memory, he quickly got his B.A. at a local community college, earned a perfect score on his LSATs, and was accepted into law school.

In contrast, a 36-year-old physician's assistant who had dropped out of medical school 15 years earlier, answered the opening inquiry with, "I need help in deciding whether or not to go back to medical school." In this case, no hidden assets became evident. The same dependency, anxiety, and ambivalence that led to his original withdrawal from school still permeated his presenting complaint, which in this case did serve as a telling hologram. Until the patient became aware of his real situation, the therapist could only stand by, ready to pick up the pieces when his efforts to regain admission misfired, as they in fact did.

A 32-year-old stock analyst presented with, "I have been seeing two different women for the past 4 years; my previous therapist said I had to come clean and tell them, but I can't do it." Here the type of splitting, permitting intensely divided loyalties, casts serious doubts on his ability to form an undivided therapeutic alliance. Therapeutic support for putting an end to his acting out has not led to meaningful change, only to the further acting out of seeking another opinion. Based on his track record, the "previous" therapist could very well be current, in which case the new therapist is being scrutinized for his willingness to take part in another triangle. Presented with the idea that his current predicament was a replay of being caught between warring parents in childhood, he seemingly agreed with the interpretation but canceled his subsequent appointments.

In an entirely different vein, a patient referred for medical psychiatric evaluation complained that "I'm still depressed, even though my therapy is winding down. It has helped me in so many ways, but bad moods still come over me for no good reason. My therapist thinks the problem might be biological." Although the patient experienced significant side effects from the prescribed antidepressant medication, he nevertheless tolerated them and achieved an excellent result: Not only did the bad moods go away, but he gained greater awareness of the psychological determinants of his depressive episodes. The presenting complaint served as a prognostic hologram of this good outcome; he expressed goodwill and gratitude toward his therapist despite an imperfect result. Thus, he experienced his past treatment as generally positive, which meant that he was likely to be kindly disposed toward his further treatment with me. Moreover, he had the blessings of his therapist, who made a positive referral for biological evaluation, and he himself showed no fear or suspicion of taking medications. Everything added up to a positive, conflict-free approach to medical-psychiatric treatment.

As the reader will see in Chapter 8, however, resistance to taking medication may seriously impede the achievement of optimal results. Negative feelings about psychoactive medication may compromise drug efficacy or enhance side effects, as it did initially in Howard's case. A history of unsuccessful past treatments is just the sort of information that the history of the present illness is designed to provide.

THE HISTORY OF THE PRESENT ILLNESS

This section of the case study is the most direct inquiry into patterns of reenactment. It starts with an attempt to document the particulars of the chief complaint. For example, Howard's presenting complaint was, "I am having trouble with women." Eliciting the present illness started with asking what kind of trouble and then went on to find out when it first started, what were the initiating circumstances, what made it better or worse, and what impact it had on the capacity to work and sustain other relationships.

Often, in such an account, the patient tells only of the most recent instance of having trouble. The key to discovering patterns of reenactment, however, is to ask the crucial three-part question: Has this ever happened to you before, what was done about it, and what was the outcome? This is the single most important question sequence in the psychiatric case study. Answering it accurately and thoroughly opens a window not only onto the patient's unconscious patterning but onto his or her potential future—that is, onto the future that would most likely evolve without the corrective influence of psychotherapy. When we discover that a patient with recurrent panic attacks has found fault with and discontinued four previous competent attempts at therapy, then we know that the prognosis for a good outcome is very poor.

In Howard's case, his most recent trouble with a woman involved a secretary at the office. She was constantly weeping because she was "in love" with him, while he kept telling her, "We have to stop seeing each other because there's no future in the relationship." His previous serious relationship, 3 years earlier, broke up in similar circumstances when the young woman declared her love for him. Most revealingly, on that occasion Howard was aware of feeling love for her until the very moment she declared her own love for him, at which time his own feelings "went dead," never to be awakened again. This sudden cutoff of feelings, of being involved in an important interaction while feeling outside it, is a crucial indicator of a reenactment in progress, originating from a prior grief-reducing dissociative split. It takes place in an altered state of dissociated consciousness.

The prototype of this "trouble with women" was Howard's relationship with his mother. At age 5, after an argument with her, he went on a hunger strike and started losing alarming amounts of weight. By this action, he rejected his mother's essential mothering function—giving food, love, and care—to the point of endangering his life. She and his father allowed Howard to get away with it, letting him take control of his own nourishment. At age 8, he angrily broke loose from his mother's alcoholic embrace; she weepily complained, "Why can't you be more loving?" These were the very scenes that were played out with his most recent girlfriends: He became involved with obviously sick women, then frostily rejected their offered love, resentfully withdrawing when love was asked from him. The girlfriend in high school appears to have been an exception in that she rejected him immediately upon his return from Vietnam, before he had a chance to withdraw.

The prognosis, then, was that Howard was apt to end up alone, because he would reject any woman who did not reject him first. Her love would be angrily refused as if it were bad milk. A woman's attempt to give him love would run into his anorectic need to overcontrol and limit his own intake. Thus, successful treatment of Howard would involve undoing this pattern by getting him to accept parental feeding and derive gratification from it. Only by doing so would it be possible for him to enjoy an intimate relationship (by definition, a mutually feeding one). Getting him to accept gifts from me, then antidepressant medication, and finally Beth's nurturant care were the crucial steps that led to his successful marriage.

Turning to Beth's present illness, I could find no childhood prototype of her drunken, arrogant, battling relationships with men, except in her competitive relationships with her siblings. The pattern seemed to be in large measure the consequence of her adult-onset manic-depressive illness, often associated with poorly tamed primitive instincts, and a lack of effective parental limits and discipline arising out of her oedipal victory. What was clearer was that, for whatever reason, her lovers were not her friends but her opponents. Thus, she was headed for a life of extremely stormy, disruptive relationships—typical of borderline patients—if medicine and limits were not successfully deployed. Only after the acceptance of external control might she then be able to take the further step of assuming self-control and thereby head off the numerous breakups looming on her horizon.

To be effective, however, the external controls would have to be applied more consistently and pervasively than intensive outpatient therapy usually affords. Instead she would have to be embedded in an extensive therapeutic milieu that provides ongoing corrective feedback beyond normal therapy time, not only from me but from Howard and her fellow group members. The staging of this kind of treatment will be discussed further in the next chapter.

We are looking at patterns of reenactment from the present illness that suggest what acting out behaviors need to be stopped in order for patients to reach their goals. Thus, as the reader has seen, Howard and

Larry were helped to stop relationship-destroying behaviors so that they could ultimately achieve intimacy. The assumption in these cases is that the goal of intimacy is feasible and attainable if self-destructive behavior can be stopped. By way of contrast, sometimes the present illness tells us that the patient's sought-after goals are misconceived and should be dropped. For example, Elena, the architect who repeatedly resigned or was fired from her jobs in reenactment of an early family banishment, continued to do poorly in institutional settings even after therapy yielded insight into the determinants of her behavior. A creative, loner type, her present illness made it clear that she should give up on finding a "job" and instead develop an individual lifework. As a private freelancer, she achieved the success and satisfaction that had previously eluded her. Now with multiple employers instead of a single one with threatening power over her, she avoided the negative transference reactions that had sabotaged her past employment. More inspired, she was able to envision projects of social significance and to get them funded. Not everyone can be a team player!

In this case and many like it, the therapist must give the patient's "watchful guardian" credit for refusing to cooperate on certain projects. Sometimes working together with the internal saboteur, the guardian sets out to block chosen tasks for which the individual is fundamentally unsuited. It helps the natural artist flunk out of medical school so that she can pursue her true work. It helps the academic perish by not publishing so that he can go into business, for which he shows great talent. In the face of overwhelming evidence of intractable patterns of reenactment, the therapist must help the patient see that certain ventures are misconceived and must be replaced by more suitable ones that lie outside the web of cruel fate. As Idries Shah puts it, there are no failures, only misconceived plans. Sometimes only by bowing to destiny do we, Houdini-like, escape its iron embrace.

THE PAST HISTORY

The past history should be an account of the patient's track record along several dimensions: general health, childhood and adult development, educational level, career trajectory, social relationships, drug history, and legal entanglements. Track records have two components: patterns of reenactment and real levels of achievement. Thus, in determining a patient's track record with respect to health, we are interested first in recurrent patterns of good or bad health, particularly in response to life events, and second, to the general level of health achieved in the intercurrent periods. Similarly, with respect to career and education, we are interested in the patterns of success and failure. Has the patient repeatedly flunked crucial qualifying examinations or always risen to the occasion and achieved higher positions? Despite these events, how well has he or she done overall in chosen fields of endeavor? Quite surprisingly, some individuals win major degrees and prizes but fail subsequently to do meaningful work, while others collect few tokens of outward success but still manage to create a valuable body of achievement.

In exploring the patient's various track records, crucial information that may have been overlooked in taking account of the present illness is often recovered, providing a much firmer basis for assessing the patient's chances for future health and happiness. For example, Howard's educational and career track records provided the necessary correctives to underestimating his chances for success in therapy. He failed the ninth grade, became truant, and did not even finish high school. But in the service, he drew on the example of fellow soldiers to pursue his education: He read a great deal on his own and passed his high school equivalency examination. He got into college, where he did poorly in his formal courses but excelled at work-study jobs. On this basis, he secured a good position after graduation and, despite being taken advantage of by his colleagues, he modeled himself on his boss and ultimately rose to the managing directorship of his firm. He was thus seen to be a poor starter who was a strong finisher, a bad-student dropout who nevertheless ended up at the head of his class. Crucial to his recovery from poor starts and bad grades was his ability to learn on his own, not from formal education, but from the examples set by others. But this is surely the key variable in profiting from psychotherapy: being able to use the therapist and fellow group members as role models for self-education.

In his love life, Howard had made a typical bad start. He had flunked out of every relationship until he began his therapy at age 35. But just as in his career, he overcame his bad record to find happiness in his private life. Once again he identified with a role model, his therapist, and allowed me to guide him and provide the social supports that he needed to form a stable marriage and family. Despite his initial reclusiveness and pattern of failed love affairs, his education and career track records held out hope that he would be able to transfer the same skills to the domain of his private life and achieve similar successes there.

Of course, a good track record in one domain hardly guarantees success in another. In many cases, patients compensate for failures in one area of their lives by becoming overachievers in another. The success there, far from being a generalizable hologram, is a symptom (albeit a productive one) of forfeited potential elsewhere. For example, a 43-year-old academic who sought help for depression and lack of love relationships had experienced great career success, achieving a tenured professorship at a local university. In this case, however, career achievement did not justify optimism with regard to intimacy. Unlike Howard, she had never sustained romance for more than a few weeks and had never lived with a man for even a few days. Nor was she at all interested in becoming intimate with a woman. Every time she became involved with someone, she found fault and soon broke the connection. Not enough insight or self-control could be marshalled to derail the pattern. In contrast, an obese psychotic woman, alone and out of work, had been previously married and had two long-standing affairs despite psychiatric hospitalizations. Moreover, when she followed a structured treatment program and took her medicine, she always in the past pulled herself together, lost weight, and found a lover and a job. She did exactly the same thing again only a few months into treatment.

What can be generalized from a track record in one domain to another is drive, persistence, and resourcefulness. For these to matter, however, one must also find rudimentary successes in the major tasks of the problematic domain. For example, if success in the work life is to have relevance for the love life, then the adult must have already demonstrated some sexual and social competence (i.e., some ability to have exclusive intercourse and intimacy for more than a few weeks). The individual who has reached age 40 without having achieved either is a very poor candidate for a good therapeutic outcome, no matter what his or her other track records show. Similarly, reaching middle age without ever holding a steady job or advancing in a career carries a poor prognosis for work success, no matter what other competencies exist.

Crossing the Line

By asking about brushes with the law, the therapist can use the past history to determine whether the patient has been caught violating the basic ethical norms of the society. Becoming addicted to cocaine or alcohol, molesting children, flashing in the park, stealing from clients, assaulting loved ones, breaking contracts and getting sued—all these involve crossing lines of behavior that ordinary therapy patients do not breach. The latter find other, more lawful ways to express their needs and allay their tensions and frustrations. For those who have crossed the line on repeated occasions, however, there is every possibility that the psychic pain generated by psychotherapy will, instead of evoking heightened self-control and redirection, cause them to cross the line again and thus effectively subvert the therapeutic process. Patients who are able to reform, who are able to come back from these journeys into hell and lead an ordered life, typically have to overcome denial by acknowledging their transgressions and then subordinate themselves to a higher discipline or authority, such as found in certain kinds of multistep rehabilitation programs. On this base, a multidimensional psychotherapy has a chance of allaying symptoms and refueling the fires of psychological healing and growth.

FAMILY HISTORY

Taking a careful family history is, first of all, important to determining whether the patient has a genetically transmitted psychiatric disorder. The therapist must ask if grandparents, parents, siblings, aunts, uncles, and cousins have ever had depression, mania, anxiety attacks, phobias, compulsions, nervous breakdowns, alcoholism, religious fanaticism, criminal tendencies, shock treatments, psychoactive medications, and so on. The answers have diagnostic and treatment implications: Not only do the underlying disorders tend to run in families, but so do the most effective modes of therapy. Therefore, interventions that have proven effective in close biological relatives are likely to work in the patient. For the modern therapist, making these determinations is a vital aspect of taking a family history.

But there is also a psychosocial aspect of the family history that has direct bearing on the conduct of psychotherapy. As already seen in the cases of Larry, Beth, and Howard, the structure of patients' relationships to parents and siblings are precisely what they reenact in the course of their interactions with partners, children, employers, and colleagues throughout the course of their lives. Prior to therapy, Howard reenacted his passive-aggressive relationship with his mother in all his adult love affairs, thereby making them most unlikely to succeed. By and large, patients tend to become intimately involved with individuals whose personalities are amalgams of their mothers' and fathers' attributes and who therefore offer the opportunity to relive the structure of original bonds. Thus, information about family relationships is vital to understanding what kind of difficulty the patient is getting into—why, for example, Howard was attracted to needy women whose expressions of love activated his rejection—and how this pattern might be changed. Sometimes these family patterns come out in the course of taking the present illness, but often they must be evoked by carefully targeted inquiry.

Thus, Beth's family relationships told me a great deal about why she had so much difficulty getting married, and why the marital bond, once formed, was so firm. As an oedipal victor, she was married to her father and had contempt for her mother. Therefore, she picked men whom she had contempt for and who therefore had no chance of displacing the father in her affections. Therapy involved introducing an authoritative father substitute (the directive, paternalistic therapist) into her life and then using his authority to embed her in a therapeutic milieu that supported her relationship to a respectable man, a worthy replacement for her father. Once she bonded with Howard, she accorded him the same intense loyalty that she had always felt for the father. In fact, in her own mind and that of her siblings, Howard was installed as the father-substitute of the extended family, as evidenced by his occupying the head chair at family gatherings. Beth's grief over her father's death, which initially drove her into therapy, was resolved by replacing him—first with an effective therapist who set limits and treated her mood and thought disorders, and second with an effective husband who performed certain fatherly functions, such as reining in her manic behavior.

As we saw in Chapter 1, Larry's family structure set him up to reenact sadomasochistic patterns. He repeatedly distanced himself from close connections to manage the anger and depression that were stirred up, feelings that his father's cruel mistreatment initially evoked. When he did not distance himself, he fell into either abusing or being abused by the women in his life (on the model of his relationship to his father) or regarding them as the pitiful victims of someone else's abuse (on the model of his relationship to his mother). All these patterns were so objectionable to his healthy mature self, however, that he repeatedly disrupted his love affairs. Elucidating these patterns was the main fruit of taking a careful family history in Larry's case.

In concluding this discussion, I will preview the topic of the next chapter, treatment planning, by showing how Larry's family history was further used to anticipate the preconditions of his successful therapy. His family history, properly interpreted, tells us something quite startling about what he needed to become successful in love and work. The fact is that Larry, for the first 18 years of his life, worked many hours each day on his isolated family farm, milking, plowing, and harvesting. He worked hard and with great dedication to make a success of the venture in which the whole family (mother, father, sisters, and brother) was intimately involved. Despite his father's cruelty, he still believed in the heartland value that the family love unit is the best economic unit, that "the family that works together stays together."

The profound effect these early years had on him was eloquently testified to by the way he looked and talked when he described his professional work. He carried about him the aura of the farmers I had known as a youngster: always worried about the weather (or, currently, the business climate); jumping up early to start the day's labor; working tirelessly, plying the phones as he once plowed the fields; describing in endless detail every stand of corn (or, now, every important client); and going to bed early in a state of emotional and physical exhaustion in search of the rest that would ready him for a similar tomorrow. What had made all these hard workdays possible in his youth was that he was doing it with and for the family.

What this meant for the present was that his current love and work life might need to be intertwined. In order for him to become happy and successful, Linda might have to join him at the office and become his "farm wife"—his work partner as well as his love partner. Prior to this arrangement he felt very frustrated, lonely, and empty at the office, and he had many ups and downs in his business, sometimes barely skirting bankruptcy. Once Linda joined him at the office and worked toward becoming his partner, the situation improved. He began to feel optimistic and supported in what he was doing. He enjoyed teaching her how to handle clients and employees and to share with her the planning, rejoicing, and commiseration characteristic of good partners. The result was that business began to pick up, and the office became a happier, more productive place. Unfortunately, they were subsequently hit very hard by an economic recession, leaving the firm's viability in doubt. But the business climate, not Larry's behavior, was the culprit now. He and Linda were doing their part.

It is very important in taking a family history to get clear not only what was bad about family relationships but also what was good enough to inspire patients to seek certain family ideals in their own lives. Helping clients become aware of these often unconscious longings and then realizing them in the real world are often the preconditions of a successful therapy and a rewarding life.

SUMMARY

In this chapter, I have looked at the principles of history taking that alert the therapist to the constructive and destructive patterns in the patient's life. I have advocated two major principles of interpretation in assessing the patient's clinical history: the theory of reenactment, and the idea of the hologram. I have looked at selected parts of the psychiatric examination and shown how these two principles can help the therapist understand why the patient's life has taken its past form and what is likely to transpire in the future, both with and without corrective changes. Most importantly, looking at holograms and patterns of reenactment can also give us clues as to what must be done to overcome self-defeating behavior and help the patient achieve the basic goals of the unified self, which are meaningful work and fulfilling love.

NOTES

1. H. I. Kaplan and B. J. Sadock, eds., *Comprehensive Textbook of Psychiatry,* 4th ed., Baltimore: Williams and Wilkins, 1985, pp. 487–499.
2. N. G. Hamilton, "A Critical Review of Object Relations Theory," *Am. J. Psychiatry 146*:1552–1560, 1989.
3. S. Freud, "Beyond the Pleasure Principle," *Standard Edition,* vol. XVIII, pp. 20–23.
4. T. Mann, "Freud and the Future," *Essays,* New York: Vintage Books, 1957, p. 312.
5. Freud, op. cit. p. 22.
6. K. H. Pribram, "The Neurobiologic Paradigm," in: C. Eisdorfer, et al., eds., *Models for Clinical Psychopathology,* New York, Spectrum Publications, 1981.
7. K. Popper, *The Logic and Scientific Discovery,* London: Hutchinson, 1959.

CHAPTER 6

Making the Diagnosis and Staging the Treatment

To the extent that different disorders require different treatments, an accurate determination of what ails the patient is the crucial first step in providing effective care. As was discussed in Chapter 3, the bio-existential viewpoint enjoins the therapist to make this a multidimensional assessment. Diagnosis in its fullest sense should give an accurate account of what is both sick and healthy about the patient at all five levels of the bio-existential hierarchy. Otherwise, the resulting therapy will have little chance of achieving comprehensiveness, of promoting not only symptom relief but psychological growth and integration.

STAGING

The first step in this process is to fit patients into the right biomedical categories of disorder, as defined by the latest diagnostic and statistical manual of the American Psychiatric Association, currently in its revised third edition (DSM-III-R). In so doing, the therapist determines whether the patient meets the criteria of an organic, affective, schizophrenic, personality, or other standard type of disorder. Depending on the outcome of this decision-making process, he or she institutes the modes of treatment appropriate to the qualifying diagnoses. As the reader saw in Beth's case, an initial mistake here—labeling her dysthymic instead of bipolar—led to the wrong choice of medication and an abortive first try at therapy. In contrast, subsequently making the right diagnoses of manic-depressive and borderline personality disorders entailed putting her on lithium, curbing her unstable and impulsive behavior, and teaching her more adaptive habits. The resulting behavioral control, the product of biomedical and behavioral interventions, provided the foundation for successfully applying the psychodynamic, social, and existential techniques that overcame her instability in relationships and allowed her to form a successful marriage.

First, I made the biomedical diagnoses and instituted the indicated psychoactive drug therapy. Next I looked at her maladaptive habits of impulsive, disorganized behavior and imposed limit-setting, response-preventing conditions on them. Then I looked at the psychodynamics of her oedipal victory and the dissociation of an internal saboteur that blocked all her attempts to sustain intimacy with an appropriate man. Subsequently, I determined that her family and friendship networks were inadequate to hold her in an intimate relationship and move it toward marriage; therefore, I supplied the missing social support by placing her in a group-based therapeutic milieu. Concurrently with all these interventions, I paid attention to the existential goal of helping Beth achieve freedom, based on developing beliefs and ideals that integrated the self and inspired continuous psychological growth.

Of course, the process was not quite so smooth as I have made it sound. There were problems in reporting and compliance that sent us on detours off the main highway of Beth's treatment. But there were no major roadblocks to roughly following the bio-existential sequence. When reviewing Howard's treatment, by contrast, we can see that the actual sequence fell considerably short of the ideal. At the outset, his symptoms did not meet criteria for a biomedical diagnosis. He was compulsively busy but not a clear-cut obsessive-compulsive; he had unstable intimate relationships but was not borderline in any other sense; he had eating rituals, but they hardly justified the label of anorexia nervosa; and though he was mildly anhedonic and socially withdrawn, he lacked the depressed affect and vegetative signs that would justify a depressive diagnosis.

Moreover, I judged it imprudent to start off by penalizing him for missing appointments or showing up late. I was certain he would quit therapy if I did. Also, he was not initially open to any but the simplest psychodynamic insights. So I quickly skipped to the social level of care, responding to his reclusiveness by placing him in a therapy group. Only after he caught hold in it and got involved with Beth was I able to go back and explore the dynamics of his childhood relationships to see how they were reenacted in the present (psychodynamic level). Later yet did I set limits on his passive-aggressive and compulsive behavior patterns (learning theory level).

Most striking of all, only near the end of his therapy, rather than at the beginning, was I convinced that he suffered from a core biological depression that should be treated by antidepressant medication. To arrive at this conclusion, I had to recognize that he had defensively altered or masked his mood symptoms so that neither of us could see them clearly. I came to understand that his neurotic work, eating, and relationship patterns were all layered on top of an early depressive reaction to maternal deprivation—no doubt a biologically predisposed reaction, given his family history of alcoholic-depressive illness—and that these personality traits involved dissociative, passive-aggressive, and compulsive defenses that served to attenuate the unbearable feeling of grief lying beneath them.

Once I became convinced of the existence of the underlying depression, I took the steps to uncover its characteristic symptoms and then to alleviate them. Getting him temporarily to cut off from his father served as the initial step in this process. Subsequently inducing him to take a gift and then an antidepressant from me (symbolically pushing an anorectic self-starver into letting himself be properly fed) served not just as a pharmacological treatment but as a multilevel, holographic repair of his core pathology.

Why did it take so long to make the biomedical diagnosis and treatment interventions in Howard's case? It happened because his core depression was split off from consciousness and buried under defensive character armor. The defensive armor had to be penetrated to reveal the underlying disorder and to provide the necessary treatment. This usually takes time, particularly if the patient has great anger and mistrust over early violations of his basic needs for nurturance and autonomy. Thus, any earlier attempt to get Howard to take antidepressants (i.e., before strong therapeutic alliances with me and group members had been forged) would likely have activated unmanageable feelings of rage and vulnerability that would have overridden any positive pharmacological benefits.

In light of this account, it is clear that the logical staging of the diagnostic and treatment process, which involves sequentially ascending the hierarchy of the bio-existential levels as recommended in Chapter 3, does not always work psychologically. Psychological defenses may make it initially impossible to discern the crucial symptoms of disorder, causing the therapist to miss the main diagnoses and therefore to misjudge the optimal interventions. Then again, many patients will not carry out the recommended medical or psychosocial regimens until their defenses are overcome and they come to trust the therapist and feel understood and appreciated by him or her in the fullest existential sense.

What I will do in the following discussion is to go over the main defensive barriers to an orderly diagnosis and treatment of depression, the most common substrate of mental and psychosomatic disorders. The following case illustrates any of the mechanisms that impede this task.

THE CASE OF HENRY AND ROZ

Henry, a successful businessman, was 56 when he first came for an evaluation for abdominal pain and swelling. He was referred by a friend who had been successfully treated with antidepressants for a "psychogenic" pain syndrome. He had a copy of the results of his recent workup at the Lahey clinic—five typed pages of slightly abnormal physical findings and laboratory data, unyielding of a clear diagnosis. He was urged, at the end of the report, to return to Boston later on, when the clinic's diagnostic capabilities would be better! This was just one of many inconclusive medical workups that Henry had undergone over the past 20 years, with the difference that he was now finally convinced that his problems were mental, not physical.

He described his symptoms as

> abdominal cramping pain and distension, sometimes hitting me after I eat, but it can come out of the blue. It's particularly bad after work at home. If I'm aggravated about something, the pain and distension can come with nausea, headache, and a surge of diarrhea. Sometimes I wake up in the middle of the night with a headache and stomach cramps, and I can't get back to sleep.

The discomfort came frequently enough that it limited his social life, and he had long ago given up traveling with his wife.

Henry admitted that his marriage was in trouble but could not initially be more specific than to indicate a great deal of bickering and sexual conflict. The couple's educational levels were highly discrepant: His wife had an advanced degree from a major university, while he had barely managed to finish high school. "She should have married a college professor. I'm just a businessman." He said she constantly nagged the children and himself.

His father lost all his money in the great stock market crash of 1929, after which he was a broken man. But Henry's feelings toward him were warm, in sharp contrast to his mother, whom he actively disliked. He implied that she told lies and always had a hidden agenda when she was nice. She did not take his side in disputes with others. He always felt terrible after he spent time with her.

In essence, then, this was a man whom was vaguely distressed and who somatized his pain. He could not, however, openly admit that he was depressed. To the contrary, he presented himself as cheerful. He was clearly an energetic person who was successful in business but not in his home life. He could not describe his own feelings, nor those of others—a disability that is sometimes called alexithymia or mood blindness. He was uncertain that his father had been depressed, despite giving ample evidence of the fact. And he was unclear about his own feelings. All he knew was that he felt bad most of the time, but as he put it: "I'm convinced it ain't my liver." My judgment was that his somatic complaints, which constituted an irritable bowel syndrome, were transient mood drops indicative of an affective spectrum disorder. His symptoms were masked, limited attacks of anxiety-depression.

Henry initially responded very poorly, however, to antidepressant medication. On 25 mg of nortriptyline, he felt "wired." On 100 mg of doxepin, he was too sedated to drive his car safely. As he reported these difficulties, there was a note of triumph in his voice: I had joined the long line of physicians who had failed to fix his problem. I suggested that his wife come in for a marital conference in the hopes of finding a clue to the refractory nature of his condition.

At the conference, Henry's wife, Roz, who was commandingly articulate, spoke of him in very derogatory terms. In his presence, she described him as an "obviously depressed and angry person who is completely unpsychological and therefore shows his feelings in physical symptoms. If he would get himself straightened out, our marriage might have a chance." Not only was the tone condescendingly intellectual, it strongly suggested that she was projecting some of her own problems onto Henry.

Caught off guard by this attack, I did not act to protect Henry or to register how deflated and intimidated he had obviously become in Roz's presence. But when he postponed his next appointment, the full import of the meeting came home to me. In the meantime, more reports of the successful antidepressant treatment of limited, physically manifested mood disturbances appeared in the literature,[1] and I realized that I had not tried major classes of medication in his case. After several weeks of waiting for him to make the promised new appointment, I wrote him a note saying that I hoped he would return, because I had learned things at the marital conference that might lead to a successful use of medication in his case.

A week later, he called, claiming that he had intended to return even without my letter but that he appreciated it greatly. At our session, he was visibly shaken when I told him that I thought his wife treated him abusively at the conference and that I had failed to defend him. He admitted that he had always felt abused and intimidated by her psychologizing and only recently begun to suspect that it was "book knowledge," not the kind of practical psychology that he drew on, for instance, in managing his employees. Emboldened by his responsiveness, I pointed out that although his symptoms were no doubt physically based, they also served a retaliatory purpose, effectively controlling (though self-destructively) the relationship with his wife and ultimately winning all previously lost arguments with her. All he had to do was say he was too sick to talk, travel, or make love.

His response was, "So you agree my stomach problems are real but that I am also passive-aggressive." Nodding, I went on to say that he could not let the medicine work for two reasons. First, he would be giving up his most potential weapon in the otherwise uneven battle with his articulate wife. Second he had always been fed a lot of poison, first by his mother and then Roz, about being in the wrong—even his gastrointestinal symptoms smacked of being poisoned—and because the medicine seemed like more of the same, he would have great difficulty in tolerating its side effects. To minimize the losses involved in getting better, I urged him to keep quite about any improvements in his condition except to me.

Henry agreed to try an MAOI antidepressant, despite my emphasizing that it could, in fact, be a poison if the dietary restrictions were violated. On 45 mg of phenelzine (Nardil), he experienced a remarkable lessening of symptoms and a greater sense of well-being. Concurrently, however, be became increasingly intolerant of Roz's judgmental, deprecatory treatment of him. In fact, he began to notice that his gastrointestinal symptoms and sleep disturbance, now much improved, tended to emerge after she had verbally attacked him in the course of a disagreement and that he was becoming aware of feeling angry and depressed about it. He urged her to come to me for a consultation in the hopes that I would straighten her out.

At the consultation, I discovered that Roz had experienced a major depression in her early adult years prior to marrying Henry and that she had self-medicated with stimulants at that time. Once she had married Henry, however, she became more unhappy with him than herself, and he developed his gastrointestinal and other physical symptoms. After giving a clear history of her past depression, however, Roz denied that it had any significance. Instead, she claimed she had been unhappy "for good reasons": her parents' inadequacy back then, and now having a husband who was "an emotional child." She said she might have to break up the marriage if he did not get better. My only intervention at this point was to stress the fact that Henry was unlikely to make major personality changes.

As I saw it, Henry's wife had dealt with her depression by getting married and projecting it onto her husband. In a reenactment of his relationship to his mother, he obligingly took the poison in (in part because of a psychobiological vulnerability) and developed masked-depressive psychosomatic symptoms, which also served a secondary retaliatory purpose. The couple had lived in this state of symptomatic warfare for 23 years. Now, however, the balance had been upset in that Henry was no longer willing to be depressed for both of them. If he continued to get better, the marriage threatened to unravel, and Roz might very well develop a major depression again. As someone who did both individual and marital therapy, it seemed advisable to see them both to resolve their marital conflict without unleashing dangerous symptoms in either of them.

The problem was that Roz gave no indication of being open to treatment of her own underlying depression and paranoid projections. Their recognition, in fact, was stoutly defended against. In her individual sessions, Roz spent most of the time telling me how well she was and how badly Henry's treatment was going. Not only was he on a dangerous MAO inhibitor, she charged, but it was no longer working. In fact, Henry was beginning to regress and to show a return of his old symptoms, despite every effort on my part to alter his regimen. With a clear tone of victory, Roz gave this parting shot at the end of one of her sessions: "You've done a lousy job with Henry. You ought to be ashamed to take his money for such treatment." Strong support on the home front!

It did not take long to figure out the cause of Henry's regression. By agreeing to treat both Roz and Henry together, I had recreated the pathogenic conditions of his neurosis: allowing his therapy to be poisoned, just as his life had been, by the involvement of his wife–mother. The holographic meaning of Henry's gastrointestinal symptoms (that he was being poisoned by his supposed nurturer) promised that he would stay sick until I decontaminated his treatment. I had to help erect a boundary to protect Henry from Roz's projected hate and despair.

To accomplish this goal, I took Roz up on her claim of wellness by discharging her from therapy—not because she was actually well, as I explained to Henry, but because she adamantly claimed to be and thereby rendered us both impotent to help her. At the same time and in an effort to concretize the change of regimen, I put Henry on a different "antidote," the MAO inhibitor tranylcypromine (Parnate). He experienced a prompt, sustained alleviation of virtually all symptoms.

I could not determine with certainty whether the change of medicine or the change in the therapeutic arrangement was the more crucial variable, because I elected to go for a symptomatic knockout by *massing* the interventions rather than trying one at a time. Getting the bad mother out of his therapy at the same time as replacing her poison with healing medication, both symbolized and actualized by the "better" antidepressant, served as a holographic as well as a pharmacologic repair of his core pathology.

Henry has done well for more than 2 years now. We have continued to meet periodically to monitor his medication and to shore up his defenses against Roz's need to project her distress onto him. In part because of his better self-defense, she reportedly became more dissatisfied with her life and sought her own therapy. She subsequently moved for a separation, which Henry accepted with appropriate resignation.

DEPRESSIVE MASKS

The common thread running through this case (as well as that of Howard) is that depression is often defensively masked, to follow Stanley Lesse's terminology,[2] and this impedes both diagnosis and treatment. Patients keep dysphoric feelings out of consciousness by a variety of defense mechanisms: in the case of Henry, by denial and somatization; in the case of Roz, by denial and abusive projection; and in the case of Howard, by dissociation and acting out. We must now look more closely at these and other common defenses to see how they influence the clinical presentation of depressed patients.

Somatization

After denial and repression, the most common mechanism for removing intolerable psychic pain from consciousness is to somatize it—that is, to take it out of the mental realm by focusing it onto bodily processes. Of course, we have very imprecise ideas about how this mind-body interaction is accomplished. What we do know is that the utilization of such a defense is in part genetically determined and in part a learned response. From the psychodynamic viewpoint, somatization is a developmentally early mode of mental pain reduction, and therefore its appearance in adult life is considered a sign of psychological arrest or regression.

According to DSM-III-R, the common somatoform syndromes are those relating to imagined bodily defects; conversion symptoms, often involving hysterical blindness, paralysis, and anesthesia; and hypochondriasis, in which minor physical symptoms are constantly interpreted as evidence of serious disease. Probably the largest group of somatized mental disorders are the psychophysiological conditions, which include several gastrointestinal conditions such as ulcer and colitis; and cardiopulmonary abnormalities like tachycardia, angina, hypertension, and asthma; and "psychogenic" pain states, particularly migraine and tension headaches and lower back and limb spasms and aches. These disorders, along with autoimmune and allergic conditions, have virtually defined the meaning of psychosomatic illness.

Although they are not properly viewed as somatoform or psychophysiological disorders, some eating, sleep, and sexual disorders should be added to this list because they too represent mental suffering spilling over into vulnerable physiological systems. As Freud pointed out, the physical symptoms may serve as concrete analogues of the mental problems—for example, the way Henry's gastrointestinal symptoms symbolized his feeling of being poisoned by his mother's nastiness, and Howard's eating rituals concretized his reproach to his parents for feeding him badly.

We now have strong clinical and research data that bulimia, narcolepsy, migraine headaches, and irritable bowel syndrome are all somatized forms of depression, for patients with these syndromes have a positive response to different types of antidepressant medication and give personal or family histories of major affective disorder.[3] Conditions in which research documentation of underlying depression is less secure but still convincing include tension headaches; anorexia; hypochondriasis; various types of neck, back, and swallowing spasms; and nonorganic pain in the back, joints, or muscles.[4] Once again, many patients suffering from these symptoms have a highly favorable response to antidepressant therapy and past histories in themselves or family members of major mood disorders.

Yet what cannot be overlooked is that those who somatize, like those who project, often have difficulty owning up to their depression and accepting medication or other depression-relieving measures, even when they work well. For example, a middle-aged paralegal with long-standing tic-like neck spasms, which she professed to hate intensely and to want removed, had a virtually complete reversal of symptoms, with a clear sense of improved spirits, on one 20 mg fluoxetine (Prozac) tablet daily. This did not prevent her from secretly and unilaterally stopping her medication and then choosing to stay off it once the deception was uncovered, despite a resurgence of both somatic and depressive symptoms!

Similarly, a compulsively cheerful biochemist with a strong personal and family history of major depression jeopardized his marriage and his health by frequent homosexual contacts. Put on an antidepressant (nortriptyline 75 mg daily), he noted complete disappearance of homosexual desire and a greater sexual and personal interest in his wife, accompanied by a clearly recognized improved mood. He stopped going to gay bookstores altogether. Yet, overriding my objections several months later, he decided to go off his medication. "It can't be good for the body to swamp it with foreign chemicals," he said. He soon resumed his promiscuous homosexual activity. What became apparent was that antidepressant medication reversed only his depression-relieving homosexual cruising but not his core emptiness of spirit, which could only be repaired (rather than quick-fixed) by finding adequate identifications and personified ideals. He was unable to invest the necessary time and effort to accomplish this goal.

Projection

In its most important sense, projection is an externalizing, transpersonal defense. It does more than merely attribute motives and attitudes to others. In favorable circumstances, involving highly influential projectors and susceptible receptors, a whole range of feelings and beliefs can actually be implanted in others. Great actors or political leaders play audiences in just this way, and hateful parents inject their children with their own depressions and conflicts. The most dramatic example is *folie à deux*, where an entire mental syndrome is transmitted from one individual to another by the mechanism of projection.

As shown in the previous case, Roz spared herself the pain of her own depressed feelings by unloading them on Henry and thereby intensifying his depression. All the while, she spoke derisively of his symptoms; and even though she professed a strong interest in his getting better, she fought against effective treatment because it deprived her projections of a receptive target. The fact that the projection process can work in this way has two important clinical implications. First, the target's depression may be refractory, despite expert biological and psychological interventions, until the projector's power is neutralized. Second, the projector's depression may be difficult to detect unless the target is brought into treatment and helped to resist being projected upon.

For example, an attractive, animated middle-aged professional woman, already "softened up" by the referring marital therapist, started her psychiatric consultation by admitting that for years she had unfairly blamed her husband for her own depression. Yet, during the rest of the interview, she appeared cheerful and denied the existence of sleep or eating disturbances or impairment in her ability to work or socialize. Unable to make a diagnosis, I suggested she bring her husband to the next session. He started out by saying that he loved her very much but was no longer willing to be her scapegoat. When asked what she blamed him for, he pointed to her feelings of inadequacy and social rejection and her difficulties in handling the children. According to him, she had been crying for days and had virtually stopped eating and sleeping.

With this revelation, the wife broke down, wept loudly, and said many self-derogatory things. Abruptly, she regained her composure and stubbornly denied that anything was wrong. She admitted to crying but said it was because her husband did not love her any more. With many false starts and compliance problems, she managed to follow an antidepressant regimen involving both medication and cognitive-behavioral techniques. It was obvious that her cooperation depended greatly on her husband's implicit threat of divorce. Even though her mood was significantly improved, she only begrudgingly admitted that she felt better. Yet her husband said she was enough changed to make it worth the effort to try to save the marriage. Subsequently, in her individual therapy, she worked on repairing her feeling of being "rotten at the core," which lay behind her need to project.

Dissociation

The mechanism of splitting or dissociation is thought to come into play only after major psychic trauma, such as being beaten or molested as a child. But what is abundantly clear is that in individuals who are highly predisposed (i.e., who have strong genetic leanings toward anxiety and depressive reactions and dissociative mechanisms), a considerably milder insult will cause a split. For instance, one client had the characteristic splitting experience—going numb and watching the interaction from outside—when his father chastised him for masturbating at age 11. He was a compulsive masturbator from that time until middle age. The previously mentioned patient who was banished to an infectious disease hospital at age 7 remembered going numb and having the sense of existing outside her own body at the very moment when her parents drove away from the hospital, leaving her behind. From that time on a part of her, with both saboteur and guardian qualities, reenacted this banishment by provoking numerous firings and angry resignations from schools, teams, camps, and jobs until she found a psychotherapy in midlife that helped her become a successful loner.

In Chapter 10, I will discuss how destructive subpersonalities are formed out of the dissociative and identification processes. What is important to recognize here is that underlying all acting-out behavior is a split-off angry, depressed subpersonality. It caused Howard to passive-aggressively withdraw from every woman, prior to Beth, who declared her love for him; and it caused Larry, every time he became intimate, to pick fights, become distant and morose, and even try to destroy his business, as he initially did when he fell in love with Linda. What this means diagnostically is that individuals who repeatedly act out patterns of self-defeat typically have an underlying, split-off depression that should be treated even if they are not overtly depressed. This is also true of patients who somatize and project their depression. No matter how cheerful they look and how well they sleep, depression is lurking nearby, and its characteristic symptoms should be unmasked.

Other Masks

In addition to being somatized, projected, split off, and acted out, depression can be displaced, reversed, compulsively ritualized, and rationalized in political or theological terms. Many of the depressed patients I have discussed initially appeared cheerful: They reversed sad feelings into their opposite. Also very common is the mechanism of displacement, which produces the social and simple phobias, such as fear of public speaking, travel, heights, pets, and crowds.[5] And we have seen how Howard fought off his depression by compulsive busyness and overwork. The important thing, once again, about all these defensive masks is that the patient may be depressed without appearing to be. We must now review how underlying mood disturbances can be unmasked.

UNMASKING DEPRESSION

In the absence of overt, characteristic signs and symptoms of mania and depression, there are three sets of findings that alert the clinician to the possibility of the diagnosis: (a) a past history of a frank depression or mania in the patient; (b) a history of mood disorder, nervous breakdown, alcoholism, or shock treatments in first degree relatives (parents, children, and siblings), which suggests a genetically transmitted vulnerability; and (c) the presence in the patient of "soft" signs of depression (low self-esteem, self-consciousness, shyness, separation anxiety, phobic fears, obsessive worrying, compulsivity, chronic pessimism, slowed thinking, and indecisiveness) or "soft" signs of hypomania (arrogance, garrulousness, intrusiveness, overfamiliarity, seductiveness, and histrionics). When any of these cues are present, the therapist can feel justified in vigorously pursuing the search for "hard" signs of mood disorder.

The search often pays handsome dividends. The therapist suddenly notices the characteristic disturbances of affect, energy, sleep, eating, and pleasure peeking out from behind the presenting mask. He or she is often surprised at how obvious and plentiful these classic signs of mood disturbance, previously hidden from view, suddenly become if one sensitizes oneself and actively researches for them. For example, the fact that Howard always woke up at 5 a.m. and took little enjoyment in eating was initially taken as evidence only of a spartan life-style. But once suspicion of an underlying depression grew stronger, these behaviors increasingly looked like symptoms—as they turned out to be, because they receded on antidepressant therapy. He began to enjoy a more varied diet and to sleep better as his depression resolved.

Sometimes the hidden depressive symptoms cannot be unmasked unless specific evocative steps are taken, such as setting limits on acting out, giving gifts that stir up the pain of past deprivations, or prescribing behaviors that cut into pockets of self-hatred. For example, one highly literate patient tried to quit therapy—an acting-out maneuver—when I gave her the novel *Love in the Time of Cholera* as a present. Persuaded to stay in treatment (i.e., with limits placed on her acting-out impulse), she promptly became suicidally depressed. In the depths of her despair she revealed that "my parents never celebrated any of my birthdays and never gave me a present in my whole life."

Similarly, an attractive woman who had poor grooming did nothing to improve her appearance after partially responding to antidepressant medication. Pushed into wearing makeup and having a new hairdo, she complained bitterly of "looking like a whore." When group members insisted that, on the contrary, she looked elegant, her defenses collapsed and she lamented for weeks how ugly, stupid, and hateful she felt—and then, how depressed and incompetent her mother had been. After a period of grieving, her residual depression cleared up, and she experienced her first periods of utter contentment.

Quite clearly, then, unmasking depression is only half the battle. The uncovered symptoms must also be treated. Patients who defend against experiencing depressive symptoms also defend against having them removed, as the cases here have repeatedly shown. To get around these defenses, holographic interventions may have to be made.

HOLOGRAPHIC INTERVENTIONS

Holograms, as the reader has seen, are powerful diagnostic and prognostic indicators. They are small pieces of behavior (e.g., selling one's art collection in order to finance therapy, or secretly stopping an effective treatment) that illuminate the patient's core pathology or basic will to health. They are parts that reflect the whole psychic set-up of an individual. Just as there are holographic diagnostic findings, there are holographic interventions—that is, therapeutic moves that repair the patient's core pathology at one fell swoop. When Carl Whitaker traded kicks with the gender-disturbed patient described in Chapter 2, the interaction had the economy and power of a holographic penetration. What was lacking was a well-prepared therapeutic context: a firm alliance and mutual understanding between patient and therapist as to the nature of the core pathology and the necessity of doing something special about it. With these in place, getting Howard to accept first a gift of a recording and then an antidepressant constituted a holographic repair of his early deprivation and the protective defenses built around it. Similarly, introducing Linda into Larry's business, once the ground had been prepared, overcame his core block both to work success and to intimacy.

Quite obviously, holographic interventions are unnecessary if standard therapeutic maneuvers, such as well-targeted interpretations or behavioral practices, do the trick. When there have been major childhood losses or abuses, however, then a great deal more is usually required to repair the damage. In such cases, the holographic correction typically involves an abrogation of standard individual therapy rules, which will be the main topic of discussion in Chapter 9. Therapists may have to give not only medications but highly personalized gifts, telephone and social contacts outside of sessions, and even disclosures about their private lives, particularly their personal experiences in overcoming mental problems. One patient would not admit that she had crippling panic attacks until her therapist confessed that she, too, once had them and was successfully treated. Another depressed client, whose mother died when she was 4, made significant strides only after I sent her to see a woman colleague who rocked her in her arms. For a while, she saw me once a week and the maternal therapist twice a week. Giving her the mother replacement was the gift she needed to get well.

One of the most dramatic holographic repairs in my experience involved Lucy, an unmarried attorney in her mid-30s who had stopped dating and replaced her contact lenses with thick glasses many years before. She spent most of her free time driving 100 miles away to visit her brain-damaged father, who had been drunk, abusive, and out of work since her childhood. The significant diagnostic hologram: Lucy, at age 8, while her mother was gravely ill at home, marched into the neighborhood bar, dragged her father out to his car, and drove him home! Just think of the many things this single act says about her character. Now, 25 years later and after paying her own way through law school, she was still taking care of him.

One year into therapy, she had resumed dating but withdrew every time she got emotionally close to a man. Exhausted by the demands of her practice, she complained to her group one night that she had to make the long trip again the next day to take her father to the doctor. She would not listen to all the heartfelt pleas of the group to find someone else to escort him. Finally, I pointed out that she was obviously married to her father and that if she could not place limits on taking care of him, she would never have room for another man in her life. After this sank in, I made an outrageous offer: If she could not find anyone else, then I would drive up to her father's home tomorrow and take him to the doctor in her place. She was to telephone me later that evening to tell me if this would be necessary.

A couple of hours later, she phoned to tell me that her aunt had agreed to transport her father. At our next individual session, she appeared radiant and unburdened. She now saw clearly how she had indeed been married to him and had bonded so strongly as his caretaker in order to banish the intolerable disappointment she felt at his inability to provide even minimal care to her and her siblings. "Would you really have driven up there?" she asked. On carefully prepared soil, the offer provided the holographic repair of the lack of parental care that had spoiled all her relationships with men. Very soon thereafter she got involved in her first deeply satisfying love relationship.

Another patient made dramatic improvements in her depressed mood when I refused to listen to any more of her dreams. Prior to that time, she had compulsively recounted two or three elaborate dreams at each session, after which she seemed more distressed, despite my interpretations, than when she began. As became clear, the dream-telling was a reenactment of repeated traumatic purges and enemas given to her by a psychotic maid during childhood. Stopping the dream vomiting and diarrhea was part of a highly unorthodox holographic repair of her violated autonomy.

In all such breaches of standard therapy practices, we must examine ourselves carefully to determine if we are guilty of countertransference acting out. The charge is justified if there are more effective interventions with fewer side effects that our own pathology prevents us from utilizing. In attempting to meet patients' needs through innovative, unorthodox methods, we as therapists cannot afford to become either defensive or self-righteous. It is not at all difficult to go off the track in the hazardous work we do, and we must always be alert to this possibility.

SUMMARY AND CONCLUSIONS

In a pluralistic psychotherapy, both the diagnostic and treatment processes are multidimensional. Determining that a patient suffers from a disorder means establishing how the patient is disordered in the biomedical, learning, psychodynamic, social, and existential senses—not just from one or two of these perspectives, but from all of them together. Similarly, giving comprehensive treatment involves making well-targeted interventions at all these conceptual levels.

Logically, the diagnostic and treatment processes should follow the hierarchical sequence of the bio-existential framework by serially addressing the following questions.

1. *At the biomedical level.* What is the nature of the patient's mental illness, and how severe is it? In particular, are there organic, mood, thought, and personality disorders following the criteria of the most recent DSM? Are the mood and thought disorders at the neurotic, borderline, or psychotic degree of intensity? Is there a history of mental illness in biological relatives? Are there compensatory biological strengths in the realm of drive and intelligence? What medications or other physiological interventions might reduce symptoms with the fewest side effects?

2. *At the learning level.* What bad habits of dysfunction has the patient learned, and what conditions trigger or sustain them? Are there offsetting good habits of optimism, determination, and discipline? What cognitive and behavioral exercises would promote more adaptive patterns?

3. *At the psychodynamic level.* How immature is the patient with respect to defenses and developmental level? What are the core conflicts, and how are symptoms and defenses layered on top of each other? Are there destructive subpersonalities that cause self-defeat and, conversely, constructive ones that promote success? Are there special ego strengths that need to be supported? What insights and corrective emotional experiences are needed to advance psychological development?

4. *At the social level.* What deficiencies exist in family relationships, friendship networks, and social commitments? What inadequacies in social skills prevent overall achievement? What are the balancing potentials for greater socialization? How might group, family, and/or milieu therapy be utilized to further this aim?

5. *At the existential level.* Has the patient lost freedom of the will and become demoralized? Is there a looming destiny that can be changed? Are there compensatory intuitive and artistic gifts? What is lacking in the belief system—or what personified ideals have to be internalized—in order to integrate the self and thereby achieve freedom and creativity? What is the possibility of generating holographic interventions for this purpose?

As is apparent, each of the five perspectives poses completely different diagnostic and treatment questions. Answering them one after another gives a rounded picture of the patient's illness and health and makes it possible to give comprehensive treatment. But the psychological needs and limitations of patients and therapists alike militate against a straightforward utilization of this scheme. Penetrating insights about what is fundamentally wrong with the patient, biologically and psychosocially, might not come into focus until far into the therapeutic relationship. Only after trust is established and character armor is penetrated will crucial facts and openings be revealed. Such revelations necessarily cause the diagnostic and treatment sequences to be revised. Thus, a certain amount of artistic improvisation is clearly necessary in providing sensitive care to complex human beings.

NOTES

1. For example, see J. F. Rosenbaum, "Limited-Symptom Panic Attacks," *Psychosomatics* *28*:407–412, 1987.
2. S. Lesse, ed., *Masked Depression*, New York: Jason Aronson, 1974.
3. J. I. Hudson and H. G. Pope, "Affective Spectrum Disorder: Does Antidepressant Response Identify a Family of Disorders with a Common Pathophysiology?" *Am. J. Psychiatry* *147*:552–564, 1990.
4. See S. Lesse, "Hypochondriasis and Psychosomatic Disorders Masking Depression," *Am. J. Psychotherapy* *21*:607, 1967; D. Blumer, "Chronic Pain as a Variant of Depressive Disease," *J. Nerv. Ment. Dis.* *170*:381–401, 1982; D. Blumer and M. Heilbronn, "Antidepressant Treatment for Chronic Pain," *Psychiatric Annals* *14*:796–800, 1984; D. P. Cantwell et al., "Anorexia Nervosa: An Affective Disorder?" *Arch. Gen. Psychiatry* *34*:1087–1093, 1977.
5. D. V. Sheehan et al., "Treatment of Endogenous Anxiety with Phobic, Hysterical, and Hypochondriacal Symptoms," *Arch. Gen. Psychiatry* *37*:51–59, 1980.

CHAPTER 7

A Grief-Based Theory of Disorder

There is nothing so practical as a good theory.[1] This is especially so for practicing psychotherapists, who often find themselves in confusing, emotionally charged situations in search of a clarifying explanation. They need a theory that sheds light on both the causes of their patients' troubles and what should be done about them. To be really practical, the theory must be simple in statement yet rich in implication, both straightforward and forward looking. And it must apply equally well to lives of quiet misery as to those of stormy chaos.

These attributes characterize the most popular psychodynamic notions. The wish-fulfillment, anxiety-reduction, and repetition-compulsion theories come immediately to mind. Each of these can be stated simply and made to apply to important realms of human suffering. Yet from the bio-existential perspective, they are seriously limited in the range of their explanatory power, particularly in light of new findings in the biology and sociology of disorders. Clearly, what is needed is a pluralistic theory of symptom formation to complement the broad accounts of diagnosis and treatment that we have explored in previous chapters.

The theory I shall propose here, already implicit in prior discussions, is that the majority of mental and psychosomatic disorders are brought on by grief. *Grief* is, to be sure, a vague term, but like *sex* and *love* it has the virtue of its defect: It can be made to carry multiple layers of meaning. Thus, it can be used as a common etiological term for each of the five bio-existential levels. In its most general sense, grief is a prodrome of depression—a collection of anxiety and depressive symptoms, typically induced by an overwhelming stress or loss, that has not yet jelled into a distinct syndrome of disorder. Thus, I will use *grief* and

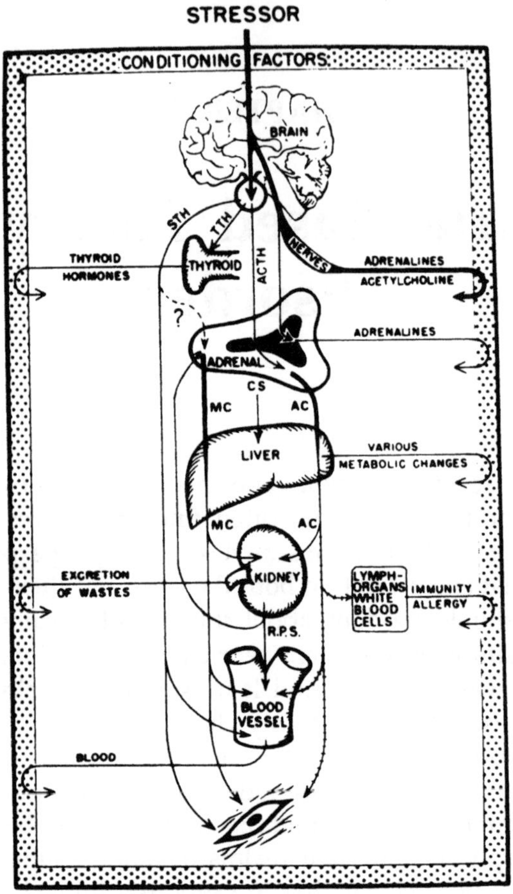

Figure 1. Selye's Atlas of Stress.

depression (in its nonspecific subsyndromal sense) as interchangeable terms.

At the biomedical level, grief is the result of traumatic stress and the chain of physiological events that Cannon and Selye first elucidated in their accounts of the fight–flight and alarm–exhaustion responses.[2] This includes sympathetic-adrenal and hypothalamic-pituitary activation, culminating in high levels of circulating norepinephrine and cortisol, which affect the major tissues and organs of the body (see Figure 1). As elucidated by Selye, arousal, if prolonged, can lead to exhaustion: thus, unregulated activation often culminates in depletion, particularly of brain norepinephrine and serotonin. From this perspective, grief-depression is the organism's manifestation of a severe, unregulated stress response; it has the psychophysiological profile of uncontrollable, overwhelming stress, to which it must be regarded as equivalent. The case for the equivalency of hyperstress and depression is strongly made by Gold et al., as summarized in Table 3.

Most importantly, this state of stress-depression creates a psychobiological environment that is highly conducive to the development, in suitably predisposed individuals, of the major psychiatric and psychosomatic disorders—and even medical ones, such as infectious and neoplastic diseases, that were not previously thought to be influenced by psychophysiological states.[3] In fact, the elucidation of the mechanisms whereby stress may lead to autoimmune and immunosuppressive processes is one of the most promising areas in contemporary medical research.[4] What must be emphasized is that from the biomedical viewpoint, whether a stress-induced grief reaction culminates in syndromal depression, dissociation, or myocardial infarction (to name just three of many possible outcomes) depends on the organism's inherited or acquired biological predispositions to these various disorders. By contrast, other biological predispositions protect those who are invulnerable from the pathogenic consequences of stress.

From the perspective of learning theory, grief results from stresses that represent a loss of control of the major reinforcements (i.e., the crucial rewards and punishments) of the individual's life. According to Seligman, such present stresses typically come in the wake of past ones toward which the individual was blocked from responding effectively, resulting in an attitude of learned helplessness. This attitude is the crucial defining quality of persistent depression or grief.[5] By operant and classical conditioning mechanisms, these pathological processes can be intensified and generalized to a range of other psychological and physical reflexes and patterns. Conversely, according to learning theory, normal, nonpathogenic grief crucially depends on the individual's past experiences of effective reparative behaviors of learned optimism.

In the psychodynamic tradition, grief results from traumatic losses of love, security, and worth. The loss of a loved one, the most devastating cause, initiates a sequence of protest-despair responses. In the course of this sequence individuals may angrily chastise either the fates or themselves but ultimately will succumb to a sense of depletion of the self. In clarifying the distinction between normal and pathogenic grief, psychodynamic theory spells out the various outcomes of the bereavement process: normal grief work leading to partial restitution; repression of the traumatic experience leading to periodic breakthroughs of conflict-anxiety; development of syndromal depression; somatization leading to psychosomatic disorders; and traumatic dissociation leading to multiple

Table 3. Parallels between the General Adaptational Response to Stress and the Syndrome of Depression

Type of Change	Stress	Depression
Redirection of behavior by the central nervous system	Acute facilitation of adaptive neural pathways	Chronic maladaptive facilitation of neural pathways
	Arousal, alertness	Dysphoric hyperarousal and anxiety
	Increased vigilance, focused attention	Hypervigilance, constricted focus, obsessionalism
	Aggressiveness when appropriate	Assertiveness inappropriately restrained by anxiety
	Acute inhibition of non-adaptive pathways	Maladaptive inhibition of neural pathways
	Decreased eating	Decreased eating
	Decreased libido and sexual behavior	Decreased libido and sexual behavior
	Appropriate caution or restraint	Excessive caution, regardless of context
Redirection of energy in the periphery	Oxygen and nutrients to the stressed body site	Oxygen and nutrients to the central nervous system
	Increased blood pressure, heart, and respiratory rates	Increased blood pressure, heart, and respiratory rates
	Increased gluconeogenesis	Increased gluconeogenesis
	Increased lipolysis	Increased lipolysis
	Inhibition of programs for growth and reproduction	Inhibition of programs for growth and reproduction
	Acute glucocorticoid-mediated counterregulatory responses (containment)	Chronic inadequate or maladaptive counter-regulatory responses (containment)
	Restraint of the corticotropin-releasing-hormone system and the pituitary–adrenal axis	Inadequate restraint of the corticotropin-releasing-hormone system and the pituitary–adrenal axis
	Restraint of the norepinephrine–locus ceruleus system	Inadequate restraint of the norepinephrine–locus ceruleus system
	Restraint of the expected immunologic or inflammatory response	Chronic immunosuppression

Note. Reprinted from P. W. Gold, F. K. Goodwin, and G. P. Chrousos, "Clinical and Biochemical Manifestations of Depression," *New England Journal of Medicine* 319:348–353, 413–420, 1988.

personality, hysteria, and other acting-out character disorders. The purpose of each of these defensive operations is to attenuate what is otherwise an overwhelming feeling of depression. Dissociative splitting is the most dramatic means of accomplishing this goal. Quite abruptly, the individual experiences a numbing relief from the pain and sometimes a discontinuity of identity and memory, even an uncanny sense of standing outside the grief experience.

From the perspective of social theory, grief is a loss of social support and connection. The death of a marital partner, which significantly increases the mortality and morbidity risks of the surviving spouse, is equally important here as in the psychodynamic tradition. But social theory also addresses the devastating consequences of losing one's larger family, group network, social status, ethnic identity, neighborhood milieu, religious membership, and national affiliation.[6] In each case, the social fabric that holds the individual's life together is torn, generating grief and the hospitable environment it provides for physical and mental disorder.

At the existential level, the stresses that produce grief and depression are demoralizing losses of meaning, brought on by seemingly mindless events that call into question the existence of a larger purpose in life. After every personal holocaust, the voice of existential grief questions the existence of a moral ledger, a higher organizing principle, in the universe. It laments the fact that the fates often appear to treat the bad and the guilty better than the good and the innocent.

In summary, traumatic grief at the biological level is the manifestation of unregulated stress, characterized by the physiological concomitants of biological depression. At the other levels, grief is the expression of a personally devastating loss of control, love, social support, and moral purpose. Injuring the person on all these planes of existence, the grief experience serves as the pathogenic substrate for most other injuries and illnesses. Even though there are congenital anomalies, metabolic errors, and chance accidents whose occurrences are not significantly stress related, what is being hypothesized is still very broad: that the vast majority of disorders is induced by traumatic losses and therefore contains a depressive core. This theory is summarized in Figure 2, which I will come back to at the end of the chapter.

Before we examine the evidence, we must ask the implicit treatment question: Does the theory imply that everyone who suffers a significant loss and becomes grief-stricken should be treated for depression? Clearly not. Human beings have natural recuperative powers; many have the capacity to heal themselves without professional help. Moreover, as many as 25% of disaster victims, who may have lost the major

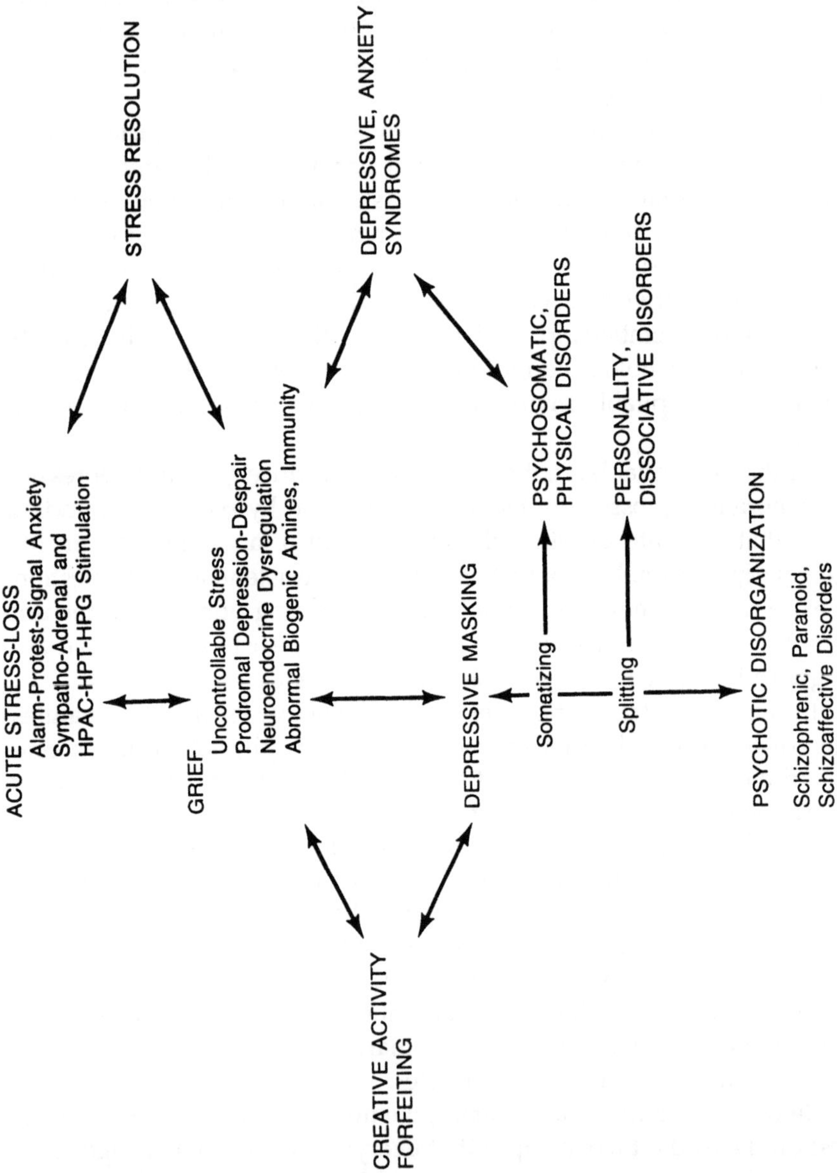

Figure 2. A grief-based theory of disorder.

sources of health and happiness in their lives, prove to be invulnerable to the pathological consequences of stress.[7] So not everyone requires treatment. But a less extreme proposal is surely recommendable: Those in danger of developing pathogenic grief should receive professional help, since the high risk of syndromal depression and other major mental and physical consequences dictates that specific preventive measures be undertaken.

At the biological level, this means a careful assessment of the feasibility of prescribing psychoactive medications and other biological interventions. From the learning theory perspective, cognitive-behavior therapy is targeted to overcoming negative thinking and replacing passive, helpless attitudes with active coping strategies. Psychodynamically, grief work involves an open exploration of positive and negative feelings about the loss and a redirection of energy in pursuit of new attachments. It may also require repair of dissociative splits and the reintegration of subpersonalities to form a whole, mature self. At the social level, efforts must be made to embed the bereaved-depressed individual in a disorder-sparing social support system. Existentially, the demoralization of lost meaning can only be overcome by the development of a new (or a reaffirmed old) belief system that makes it possible to bear the loss and to move toward freedom.

The considerable problem of knowing when the grief experience is likely to become pathogenic and therefore to require professional management is a matter of refined clinical judgment. Protracted duration and severity of the prodromal depression—melancholic features are the most serious danger signals—and a past history of grief-induced pathology should work as strong prods to therapeutic activism. In any case it is far better to overreact than underreact to the grief state, for the former can have tragic consequences, whereas the latter rarely leads to irreversible side effects.

IMPLICATIONS OF GRIEF THEORY

To say that most mental and physical accidents and disorders are triggered by stress-grief-depression is a seemingly straightforward hypothesis that is amenable to empirical testing. As the reader will soon see, however, the available evidence is spotty and needs to be filled out by further research. To begin evaluating what there is of it, we must draw out the main clinical implications of the theory. They are as follows:

1. Despite outward appearances, most mentally ill patients are in some basic sense depressed or grief-stricken and should be treated for it.
2. Most physically ill or injured patients are also depressed and could profit from medical and psychosocial antidepressant treatment.
3. Since grief is the substrate for most mental and physical disorders, their natural history typically involves a prodromal phase of stress-depression.
4. Successful treatment of most mental and physical disorders will expose the substrate of grief and thereby evoke transient depressive symptoms.
5. If severely grief-stricken individuals are caught early and given broad antidepressant treatment, the pathogenic consequences of stress will be attenuated.

These are, of course, controversial ideas, but they are testable hypotheses for which there are already relevant data. Let us see what findings are currently available and what work remains to be done.

1. *Most mentally ill patients are depressed and should be treated for it.* With regard to psychotherapy patients, this is almost a truism. Adults do not voluntarily ask for psychological help unless they have suffered a major loss or blow to independence and self-esteem. If they are honestly seeking care, they are admitting to a degree of failure, impotence, and helplessness that is equivalent to depression.

But the more important question is whether most mentally ill individuals, in therapy or not, are clinically depressed. Clearly those who qualify for the standard depressive diagnoses—manic-depressive disorder, major depression, and dysthymic disorder—fall within this category. According to epidemiological studies, the period prevalence rate of mental illness is 15% of the population, and average rates for major depression, dysthymia, and manic episodes are approximately 2.5%, 3%, and 0.5%, respectively (see Table 4). The largest remaining group consists of those suffering from anxiety disorders, which include phobias, panic attacks, and obsessive-compulsive disorder, with approximate average prevalence rates of 7%, 0.5%, and 1.3%, respectively. If we accept the evidence that the anxiety states are variant forms of depression (i.e., are subtypes of affective spectrum disorder), then our case has been made: The vast majority of the mentally ill are suffering from depression.

As the reader has already seen, patients with panic, phobic, and obsessive-compulsive disorders respond positively to different types of

Table 4. Point Prevalence Rates for Selected DSM-III Disorders, NIMH Epidemiologic Catchment Area Program

Disorder	Rate per 100 Community Residents New Haven (n = 3004)	Baltimore (n = 3058)	St. Louis (n = 3481)
Schizophrenia	0.66	0.79	0.54
Manic episode	0.53	0.38	0.60
Major depressive episode	2.55	1.79	2.64
Dysthymia	3.17	2.13	3.83
Phobias	5.13	11.09	4.04
Panic Disorder	0.37	0.65	0.59
Obsessive-compulsive disorder	1.20	1.69	1.12
Alcohol abuse or dependence	3.03	4.19	2.03
Drug abuse or dependence	1.05	1.42	1.48
Cognitive impairment (mild)	4.12	5.53	5.85
Cognitive impairment (severe)	1.20	1.28	1.00
Antisocial personality	0.32	0.52	0.80

Adapted from D. A. Regier and J. D. Burke, Jr., "Quantitative and Experimental Methods in Psychiatry," in H. I. Kaplan and B. J. Sadock, eds., *Comprehensive Textbook of Psychiatry*, 4th ed., Baltimore: Williams and Wilkins, 1985, p. 310.

antidepressant medications, have high comorbidity rates of major depression, and high incidence of major depression in family members.[8] These facts argue for a strong biogenetic connection between anxiety disorder and depression. Most importantly, the association is borne out clinically. Working over time with panicky, phobic, and obsessive-compulsive patients often uncovers the dejected feelings lying beneath their presenting symptoms, which therefore can reasonably be construed as depressive masks.

Similarly, a wide array of other mental and psychosomatic conditions meet either research or clinical criteria for depressive spectrum disorder. The evidence is particularly strong for bulimia, attention deficit with hyperactivity, narcolepsy, migraine headaches, and irritable bowel, as Hudson and Pope have shown. Other syndromes that frequently but less reliably respond to antidepressant therapy are anorexia nervosa and post-traumatic stress disorder,[9] and a whole range of hypochondriacal and psychosomatic pictures, typified by tension headaches and chronic pain states.[10] In fact, it was the existence of the last group that led Stanley Lesse to coin the term *masked depression*.

Moreover, clinical and research experience suggests that the addictions (which include substance abuse and compulsive gambling) and the severe personality disorders (which include acting-out borderline, histrionic, and narcissistic pictures) also fall on the depressive spectrum.[11] But again, the inconsistent response of these patients to antidepressants (due in part to psychological resistances, as I have shown and will discuss further in the next chapter) casts some doubt on the closeness of the presumed association. Yet, as we saw in the cases of Larry in Chapter 1 and Howard in Chapter 4, both of whom had split-off, acting-out subpersonalities, putting a stop to their acting out unmasked an underlying depression and allowed it to be successfully treated. And many addicts, when forced to become abstinent, fall ill with depression that responds to antidepressant therapy. They often tell us that their drug taking was initially an attempt to fight off depressed spirits.

Because we possess a safe, effective antidepressant treatment technology—and one that works in affective, anxiety, eating, sleep, sexual, addictive, borderline, and psychosomatic disorders—there seems little reason not to deploy it widely when criteria are met for these overt or masked affective and affective-spectrum disorders. What is not so clear is what to do with cases of presyndromal grief before pathogenicity becomes evident, and what to do with masked depressives who resist treatment of any kind despite potentially life-threatening consequences. One aspect of this latter problem, medication resistance, is the main topic of the next chapter.

2. *Most physically ill or injured individuals are depressed and should be treated for it.* There is little disagreement that depressive symptoms are common in the medically ill. According to a recent review of the literature, 12% to 36% of medical outpatients are depressed, and of medical inpatients about one-third have depressive symptoms and one-quarter syndromal depression.[12] Although very high, these figures fall considerably short of encompassing the majority of medical patients. One possible explanation is the insensitivity of our current diagnostic measures, particularly with respect to subsyndromal and hidden forms of depression. Even so, the rates are impressive in certain medical conditions. For example, as many as 50% of postmyocardial infarction patients are depressed, and 70% of them remain depressed after 1 year, a finding highly correlated with a past history of depression and subsequent psychosocial morbidity. After coronary bypass surgery, 75% of patients are reported to be depressed, and 50% of poststroke patients have depressive symptoms, with 25% having major depression. Others with high rates are patients with cancer, multiple sclerosis, Parkinson's disease, hip fracture, and endocrine disorders.

The usual interpretation of these findings is that medical conditions are quite understandably depressing, because they represent major stresses and losses of physical competence and integrity. In addition, some disease processes (e.g., abnormalities of the thyroid, adrenal, and pituitary glands) may mimic some of the chemical irregularities of biological depression and therefore reproduce its psychobiological symptoms. The standard psychiatric formulation of such findings is that depression is a "psychobiological final common pathway."[13] But what the grief-stress hypothesis implies is that depression is also an *initial* common pathway, a nonspecific precondition of disorder analogous to the inflammatory response. In other words, it predicts that depression, perhaps in a hidden form, comes first: that most medical illnesses are not only grief inducing but grief induced, a possibility I will examine in the next section.

As to the present hypothesis, much more evidence will have to be gathered to support the notion that most physical conditions are associated with depression. Much the same holds for demonstrating the efficacy of antidepressant treatment in reducing the physical and the psychosocial morbidity of physical illness. Jana Mossey and associates are currently pursuing this important area of research; they have shown that hip fracture patients with persistent depressive symptoms (20% of a total sample of 196) show poorer physical recovery than matched nondepressed patients—a strong argument for giving them antidepressant therapy.[14] Yet the sporadic positive reports of antidepressant treatment in poststroke, chronic pain, cardiac, and cancer patients[15] do not at present add up to a conclusive endorsement of this hypothesis.

3. *Most mental and physical disorders are not only succeeded but also preceded by depression.* The general theory that stress-grief is the substrate for most other mental and physical disorders at the least implies that they will have a high depression comorbidity rate. We have looked at these expected correlations in the preceding two sections. But the theory goes further and predicts that stress-depression, as a causal substrate, temporally precedes other syndromes of disorder. In the past, this was generally recognized only in connection with psychosomatic and hypochondriacal complaints. Medical and psychiatric practitioners alike have long appreciated that anxiety and depression could present as "psychogenic" physical pain and dysfunction (often called depressive equivalents) and could even amplify the symptomatology of "real" physical illness. What is being hypothesized here is the more radical claim that, with obvious exceptions, most physical as well as mental disorders are *biopsychogenic;* moreover, their antecedent biopsychogenic condition is stress-grief-depression.

To make the case for this hypothesis, one would have to show that grief or depression commonly precedes other syndromes of disorder. This would involve carefully controlled prospective studies, which are not generally available. What we have instead is suggestive research about the health consequences of stressful events. Most important among these are the investigations of Holmes and Rahe, and Paykel,[16] which attempt to quantify stressors in terms of pathogenicity. (See Table 5 for a list of the stress intensities of various life events.) This body of research strongly supports the notion that stresses and losses are the antecedent conditions of most physical and mental illnesses and injuries, but it does not show that those who have suffered these untoward life events are in fact depressed or grief-stricken as a result. From the bio-existential standpoint, as outlined earlier, this is a reasonable assumption, but it needs scientific proof.

Other studies bearing on this issue are Engel's work, which concludes that grief—of what the author calls the "giving up, given up" complex—precedes the onset of illness in 70% to 80% of all patients.[17] To be sure, this exhausted, demoralized state of subsyndromal depression can result not only from actual losses and traumatic events but from threatened and symbolic ones in suitably predisposed patients. This last point serves to remind us that the grief hypothesis is predicated on a theory of variable biological predisposition, ranging from endogenous conditions (in which no external conditions are favorable enough to spare a disorder) to states of invulnerability (in which no stressor is noxious enough to cause one).

Most physicians and behavioral scientists have little trouble in acknowledging the stress-loss precipitation of the majority of mental breakdowns, but the findings on physical illness are more difficult to accept. A study such as Schmale's, however, provides suggestive evidence.[18] In this investigation, 31 of the 42 patients admitted to a general medical service with the whole range of medical diagnoses experienced the onset of illness within 1 week of a significant loss, and 39 of the 42 became ill within 1 month of a loss. This loss-precipitation has now been established for the onset of anorexia-bulimia, autoimmune diseases, bronchial asthma, malignancies, diabetes mellitus, peptic ulcer, leukemia, thyrotoxicosis, essential hypertension, congestive heart failure, myocardial infarction, abdominal pain, ulcerative colitis, tuberculosis, complications of pregnancy, postpartum depression, and the major psychiatric illnesses.[19] Similarly, as Mossey and associates have shown, 84% of chronically depressed hip-fracture patients were depressed by history before their injury.[20] Moreover, recent widowers, the highest risk group for grief-depression, have a 40% higher mortality rate than married men of

Table 5. The Holmes–Rahe Social Readjustment Scale

Life Event	Mean Value
1. Death of spouse	100
2. Divorce	73
3. Marital separation	65
4. Jail term	63
5. Death of close family member	63
6. Personal injury or illness	53
7. Marriage	50
8. Fired at work	47
9. Marital reconciliation	45
10. Retirement	45
11. Change in health of family member	44
12. Pregnancy	40
13. Sexual difficulties	39
14. Gain of new family member	39
15. Business readjustment	39
16. Change in financial state	38
17. Death of close friend	37
18. Change to different line of work	36
19. Change in number of arguments with spouse	35
20. Mortgage over $10,000	31
21. Foreclosure of mortgage or loan	30
22. Change in responsibilities at work	29
23. Son or daughter leaving home	29
24. Trouble with in-laws	29
25. Outstanding personal achievement	28
26. Wife begins or stops work	26
27. Begin or end school	26
28. Change in living conditions	25
29. Revision of personal habits	24
30. Trouble with boss	23
31. Change in work hours or conditions	20
32. Change in residence	20
33. Change in schools	20
34. Change in recreation	19
35. Change in church activities	19
36. Change in social activities	18
37. Mortgage or loan less than $10,000	17
38. Change in sleeping habits	16
39. Change in number of family get-togethers	15
40. Change in eating habits	13
41. Vacation	13
42. Minor violations of the law	11

Note. From T. H. Holmes and R. H. Rahe, "The Social Readjustment Scale," *Journal of Psychosomatic Research* 11:213–218, 1967.

the same age.[21] Although no one of these findings is conclusive, the overall pattern has considerable weight.

With regard to mental illness, grief is clearly the stimulus for anxiety and depressive reactions, but also for most of the other major psychiatric illnesses, including psychotic reactions. Despite our nosological fastidiousness, which tries to keep schizophrenic and affective disorders entirely distinct, clinical experience teaches us that they often come mixed together; that is, the major mental disorders are frequently schizoaffective. For example, in reviewing the classic literature on the schizophrenic syndromes (e.g., Kahlbaum's work on catatonia and Meyer's on dementia praecox[22]), I was struck by the regularity with which illustrative cases show preliminary subsyndromal depressive or manic-depressive pictures, followed then by catatonic, hebephrenic, and paranoid schizophrenic symptoms. The following case from my practice is illustrative.

A college junior showed dejected mood, loss of appetite, disturbed sleep, and inability to do homework after being rejected by his girlfriend. He dropped out of school and moved back home. As he became obsessively involved with bodybuilding and exercise, his depressed mood improved considerably, but relief was only temporary. His eyes began to "wander," as he said: "They split around buildings and were drawn up into airplanes flying overhead or were pulled through keyholes by passing cars." His evident schizophrenic symptoms had been preceded by equally obvious signs of grief-depression.

The implication of such findings is that because patients often get depressed before becoming psychotic, they should be treated for their underlying depression as well as their overlying psychotic symptoms. This is also true when the salient presenting symptoms involve panicked, agoraphobic, anorexic-bulimic, addictive, borderline, and other acting-out behavior patterns. These cannot be optimally treated without concurrent attention to the accompanying depressive substrate. Much the same should be said for paranoid, schizoid, and schizotypal personality: Treating the subpsychotic thought disorders of these conditions is, in my experience, rarely completely successful without concurrent attention to the underlying grief.

4. By exposing the substrate of grief, successful treatment of mental and psychosomatic disorders will often precipitate a transient depressive reaction. As is well known, recovery from psychosis is often punctuated by the emergence of depression. Elvin Semrad, whose unique gifts as an interviewer I discussed in Chapter 2, was a pioneer researcher into these phenomena.[23] The high incidence of postpsychotic depressions is now widely recognized.[24] From the psychodynamic perspective, the emergence of these depressive symptoms represents a grief reaction to the loss of psychic integrity involved in becoming psychotic. From the biomedical perspective, however, acute psychoses are always schizoaffective, that is, mixtures of schizophrenic and affective features. Therefore, in the absence of antidepressant therapy, treatment of the schizophrenic symptoms should highlight the residual depression, which it often does.

But the grief-substrate hypothesis goes beyond predicting that grief-depression will be a consequence of recovery from psychosis. It says that the removal of a wide range of mental and psychosomatic symptoms will precipitate a grief reaction. As the overlying, presenting symptoms are suppressed or resolved, the underlying depression will be exposed. We have a wealth of clinical experiences to support this notion. For example, when Larry's acting-out personality disorder, discussed in Chapter 1, was interfered with (i.e., when he was prevented from running away from intimacy), he became clinically depressed and had to be started on antidepressants. Once Howard (see Chapter 4) broke off his hostile-dependent, passive-aggressive relationship to his father, he also succumbed to grief-depression. Paradoxically, the successful use of antidepressants in his case initially led not to improved spirits but to a period of mourning over his love-deprived childhood. The regularity with which antidepressant treatment, both biological and psychosocial, causes an initial intensification of depressed feelings provides us with a cautionary maxim: Present relief unmasks past grief.

Similarly, when we succeed in getting addicts to practice abstinence, they often "crash" into major depression. Sometimes this happens even if they are given concurrent antidepressant therapy. Should the resulting depression not be quickly resolved, the prognosis is very poor indeed for continued abstinence. In fact, if addictive behavior is not replaced by far better "antidepressants" than alcohol or cocaine—not just better medicine, but better beliefs and relationships—then recovery is likely to be doomed, as it was for the addictive homosexual cruiser mentioned in the last chapter.

Thus, if compulsive gamblers, womanizers, workaholics, shoppers, cruisers, mutilators, ascetics, or overeaters are stopped from acting out, they often become deeply depressed and require broad-gauged antidepressant therapy. If treatment is withheld or proves ineffective, the patient often feels compelled to act out again. What is being exposed is, to be sure, conflict-anxiety, as classical psychodynamic theory postulates. But at a deeper level, what comes out is *original grief*, the split-off core depression of early trauma and loss. Having been uncovered, it must now be assuaged if the patient is to be dissuaded from splitting, acting out, ritualizing, somatizing, projecting, or fragmenting again and instead helped to integrate and ascend to more highly developed modes of mental functioning. In Chapter 10, I will look more closely at how the exposure of original grief is essential to repairing dissociative splits in the self and thereby overcoming acting-out character pathology.

5. *If grief is treated early, its pathogenic consequences will be prevented.* We have virtually no controlled studies that throw light on this most important practical consequence of the grief-substrate theory. We do know from epidemiological studies that various forms of social support have beneficial effects on global mental health, recovery from depression, physical symptoms, and all causes of mortality.[25] But specific intervention studies, which treat overstressed, grief-stricken, and depressed patients early on and then measure the consequences for general health, are only now being undertaken. My colleague Jane Mossey is a pioneer in this line of work. Until these studies are completed, we have to content ourselves with clinical experience pointing to the improved mental and physical health of those who are successfully treated for grief-depression. Our unmistakable impression is that over time they get comparatively fewer colds, heart attacks, infections, and other stress-related illnesses. If such clinical findings are supported by controlled research, then the strongest possible case would be made for launching primary prevention programs in the bereaved-depressed population.

THE MEANING OF GRIEF AND ITS PERVASIVENESS

Before summarizing the various facets of this theory, we must address its fundamental supporting fact: Grief and depression are so widespread as to be virtually universal accompaniments of life. Given the precarious nature of human existence, practically no one can escape suffering major stresses and losses and the resulting states of grief. Of course, not all develop a full-blown anxiety or depressive syndrome, but all except the true invulnerables are likely to succumb to subsyndromal depressions, usually on repeated occasions, during the course of their lives. The question we must now ask is why this should be so. Neither our survival nor our biological evolution requires that we be subjected to the intense mental suffering of depression; surely an intense burning in the stomach would serve just as well to warn us of approaching dangers or to induce us to correct our past errors of judgment. What, then, is the meaning of grief and its pervasive occurrence in human affairs?

What great enough purpose does it serve to have been naturally selected by the evolutionary process?

Obviously, we can only speculate about the answer. What seems likely to me is that grief and depression are major raw materials and propellants of psychological evolution. Not just happiness and success but psychic pain and experiences of loss are what fuel advances in awareness and their culmination in enhanced moral sensitivity and artistic creation. Grief transformed provides the basis of increases in empathy, spirituality, and creativity. Our losses sometimes induce the birth pains of heightened consciousness. Without grief, we would have less potential for psychological development. Coming to terms with our repeated separations and failures demands of us that we stretch toward a broader, more universal understanding of the vast forces that shape our destiny and the limited powers of our individual minds.

Needless to say, the pain of depression does not always lead directly to either wisdom or heroism. It may instead make cowards of us all, at least temporarily, by overwhelming our capacity to cope. Initially, we may have to deaden the pain by splitting it off from consciousness, awaiting a future time when we can summon up the strength to master it. In more dire circumstances, we may even have to renounce our feelings permanently, in the process forfeiting our potential for expanded awareness and expression.

Thus, the grief experience is a crossroads from which several paths lead. The preferred one is the road of heightened psychological growth and its richest fruits, freedom and creativity. If they are legitimate products of the grief experience, then we would expect the most creative individuals to show heightened vulnerability to depressed moods. As it turns out, the evidence is quite strong. Andreasen has studied the successful writers who participated in the Iowa Writers Workshop over a number of years and discovered that 80% had depressive disorders.[26] Corroborative evidence also comes from the Harvard studies of creativity.[27] And our clinical experience bears this out: Blocked creative types, with their underlying depressions, are major seekers of psychotherapy. Rank said the neurotic is the *artist mangué*. I would revise this to say that the depressive is the potential artist.

THE STAGES OF SYMPTOM FORMATION

Having considered the pervasive nature of depression and its appearance as prodrome and "postdrome" of other disorders, we are now in a position to examine a clinically elaborated formulation of the grief substrate theory. The model envisions several main stages of symptom formation, as outlined in Figure 2. First, the individual is subjected to major stress or loss, exciting a response of alarm, signal anxiety, and protest, which can in ordinary circumstances lead to the kinds of effective actions that promote stress resolution. If the stress proves uncontrollable or exhausting, however, as evidenced by sympathetic and hypothalamic-pituitary dysregulation, then the second stage of grief and despair develops. This subsyndromal depression may also, in time, resolve itself without further pathological consequences.

Quite often, though, it serves as the substrate for subsequent mental and physical symptom formation. Depending on the psychobiological predisposition of the individual, grief may lead into a full-blown anxiety or depressive syndrome, or it may be attenuated by defensive masking. The two main forms of masking are somatizing and splitting. Somatizing can lead not only to the standard psychosomatic illnesses but to all the other forms of stress-related physical disorders mentioned earlier. Splitting typically leads to dissociative, borderline, and other severe character pathology, but it may also lead either to unconscious creative activity or to forfeiting of potential.

The narcissistically injured child or adolescent splits off the unbearably hurt part of the personality, which can become a self-defeating, disavowed primitive self. Or he or she may split off a creative higher self, operating outside of conscious control and awareness. In the form of an angry, impulsive, or harshly judgmental internal saboteur, the split-off self develops a dissociative or acting-out personality disorder, often characterized by compulsively addictive, self-destructive behavior. As part of a higher self, the hurt may serve as the stimulus and raw material for advanced, protective awareness and achievement. If the dissociative process is unavailable or fails to ward off unbearable pain and pressure, however, then the self may either forfeit (i.e., radically renounce) its potential for expression or shatter and undergo psychotic disorganization, thus entering the final, most damaging stage of symptom formation.

What we must look at now is how the various bio-existential traditions relate to the model. Because it is fundamentally a defense-utilizing theory, the model is psychodynamic at its core. It regards pathology as a layering of symptoms and defenses, so that every stage is both a defense against an unwanted state of affairs and a pathological symptom of defensive action. Thus, the first stage of alarm-protest represents both a consequence of external danger and a defense against it. The second stage of grief-depression is both a symptom of prolonged signal anxiety and also a defense against fragmentation anxiety and psychotic regression.

Similarly, somatizing and splitting can be regarded both as defenses against experiencing depression and psychosis and as symptoms of depression. Finally, psychosis itself, from this psychodynamic perspective, is both a defense against and a symptom of depression. This last point explains why some psychotics resist being reorganized: They do not want to feel again the full force of the depressive pain that their personality disorganization has partially relieved.

Because the central stage in this model is the development of grief or subsyndromal depression, which serves as the substrate for other disorders, a psychodynamically informed psychotherapy aims to remove depressive masks and by-products (e.g., by setting limits on acting out and reversing psychosomatic symptoms) while concurrently repairing the exposed underlying depressive substrate. In this task, the biological, behavioral, social, and existential approaches can all be made to serve as valuable components.

While recognizing the existence of common biological substrates responding to broad-spectrum agents like the tricyclic antidepressants, biological psychiatry nevertheless assumes that each distinct syndrome has a distinct biological profile that responds optimally to more narrowly targeted, specific agents. Thus, although all masked and overt depressions might respond to a nonspecific agent like nortriptyline, the obsessive-compulsive form of affective spectrum disorder might respond best to a more specific agent like fluoxetine or clomipramine, whereas the panic-disorder form might respond best to an MAO inhibitor. Similarly, the learning and social approaches would be utilized to alter the conditioning factors and social matrices that generated pathology in such a way that greater health and growth are promoted. By contrast, the existential approach concerns itself with more abstract issues, such as the role of failed belief systems, lost moral integrity, and thwarted creativity in producing symptoms, and how regaining these at a higher developmental level can lead to freedom and creativity.

EXPLANATORY POWER OF THE GRIEF-SUBSTRATE THEORY

Regarding grief or subsyndromal depression as a substrate for most mental and physical illnesses makes sense of several puzzling but commonly observed phenomena. It explains why antidepressant and mood-stabilizing medications are so widely effective throughout the whole range of mental and psychosomatic syndromes, and why so many different illnesses have concurrent clinical, family history, and laboratory findings of depressive disorder. Moreover, it explains why most illnesses and injuries have prodromes of stress-grief and why their postsyndromal or recovery phases are punctuated by depressive episodes. According to the theory, depression is not only a final common pathway but an initial common pathway of most disorders. The theory also sheds some light on the frequent admixture of mood and thought disorders in both borderline and frank schizoaffective disturbances.

Furthermore, by calling attention to the reversibility of these pathological processes (note that most of the arrows in Figure 2 are bidirectional), the theory predicts that recovery not only from psychosis and life-threatening physical illnesses but also from the other masks and byproducts of depression—the anxiety, eating, attention deficit, addictive, psychosomatic, and acting-out personality disorders—will lead to an unmasking of the depressive substrate. Therefore, all effective therapies, whether biological, psychosocial, or existential, will typically precipitate episodes of painful grief as part of the recovery process. Moreover, because grief is the basic issue in most disorders, interfering with the masking process (as in setting limits on acting out and thereby precipitating a depressive episode) is a crucial healing step, not an unwanted side effect, in most well-managed therapies.

Finally, the theory cuts deep into man's existential being by recognizing the intimate connection between depression and the development of the highest human potential, represented by moral sensitivity and existential freedom and creativity. Depression is not only a substrate for disease but also for advanced achievement. Thus, there is a nonpathological, as well as pathological, axis along which depression can play out. As the reader will see in the final chapter, one end of this axis is occupied by freedom, creativity, and wisdom; the other end is occupied by forfeits of sexuality, volition, and moral purpose. In forfeiting potentials and constricting the personality, we have the means of avoiding depression by limiting the range of our needs and aspirations. At our fullest and most complete, however, we can make of our grief something creatively and existentially meaningful.

This theory accords the central role to depression in all human symptom formation. In so doing, it revises and supplements psychoanalytic and learning theory, both of which give anxiety the central role. Rather than discounting the role of pathological anxiety, the theory regards it not as a primordial symptom but as one of the main modes of suffering grief, which can take anxious, dejected, or bipolar forms. This emphasis accords better with Janet's contributions and recent developments in ego and self psychology, which recognize that not all mental symptoms are attributable to psychological conflicts and signaled by the presence of anxiety. Rather, the most important ones come from deprivation and lead to depression. On a vulnerable biological base, lack of attention and caring in childhood (or loss of a key relationship at any age) results in a highly predictable sequence of responses: first, alarm and protest, which if prolonged may lead into agitated or bipolar depression; and then, as hope and resistance are given up, the onset of quiet, helpless despair, the crucial sign of retarded depression.

In any of its modes, depression or grief weakens the foundation of the whole edifice of human health. It is the original crack in the foundation that may cause the whole structure to crumble. In the weakened state of depression, patients can no longer effectively hold their ground in the battle against disorder. They develop a major mental or physical illness or suffer dissociative splitting, which pushes them into self-destructive acting out, typified by borderline character pathology. Yet those relentlessly in search of growth and health can overcome these devastating consequences by finding adequate therapeutic help to repair the dissociative splits and their underlying core depression. In so doing, they can develop an integrated self and find creative and existential meaning in their lives.

In his famous paper on neurasthenia, Freud broke through the psychosomatic crust of cardiac neurosis to find its basis in anxiety.[28] This was a great advance in the scientific understanding of the mind-body relationship. Freud provided a means of treating bodily symptoms by resolving the psychological conflict-anxieties underlying them. He showed that anxiety lies below the surface of physical and mental pathology. But beneath the layer of anxiety and its originating conflicts, late twentieth-century psychiatry has unearthed the more fundamental layer of grief-depression and its originating biological and psychological deficits. In doing so, it has revised therapists' healing role. They can no longer be content with providing the kinds of explanations that lead to conflict resolution; they must also make good on the missing biological, psychosocial, and existential lacks. To do so, they must not only be parentally directive at times but personally present and giving.

At the end of the nineteenth century, Freud saw mental illness chiefly in terms of conflicts and acts of repression that were fundamentally inescapable. The healthy individual had no choice but to live with the discontents that were the inevitable price of civilization. But this was in itself a depressed view of human potential. Freud was himself the product of a finite, absolutist age that was just freeing itself from the struggle for survival and that had not yet conceived of the unlimited energy that nuclear and psychic fusion would afford. He showed the effects of the splits and repressions (e.g., his philosophic reductionism, belied by his own creativity and rejected by the worldview of modern physics) that are so intimately bound up with the antispiritual stance of his life and work. Both in his own self-analysis and in the psychoanalysis that he bequeathed to us, he accepted the tragic voids in existence rather than holding out hope for filling them.

A few generations later, even after Auschwitz and Hiroshima, we can profit from Freud's discoveries by setting a loftier goal than he envisioned: not just resolving old conflicts by renunciation but finding new meaning by achieving freedom and creativity. With a greater sense of confidence and worth, we can set and sometimes reach a more advanced goal than conflict-free maturity based on forfeiting. We can strive for an unending evolution of consciousness.

NOTES

1. This aphorism has been attributed to psychologist Kurt Lewin.
2. Selye has summarized his life's work on stress in *The Stress of Life* (New York: McGraw-Hill, 1984, revised edition). His original pathbreaking report bears the knotty title of "A Syndrome Produced by Diverse Nocuous Agents," *Nature* (London) *148:*84–85, 1936. Cannon's work is summarized in W. B. Cannon, "Stresses and Strains of Homeostasis," *Am J Med Sci 189:*1–14, 1935.
3. Herbert Weiner, "The Concept of Stress in the Light of Studies on Disasters, Unemployment, and Loss: A Critical Analysis," in M. R. Zales, ed., *Stress in Health and Disease,* New York: Brunner/Mazel, 1985.
4. The following references give a rounded picture of our current understanding, of the influence of stress and depression on immune function: J. R. Calabrese et al., "Alterations in Immunocompetence during Stress, Bereavement, and Depression: Focus on Neuroendocrine Regulation," *Am J Psychiatry 144:*1123–1124, 1987; J. K. Kiecolt-Glaser and R. Glaser, "Psychological Influences on Immunity," *Psychosomatics 27:*621–624, 1986; and M. Irwin et al., "Life Events, Depressive Symptoms, and Immune Function," *Am J Psychiatry 144:*437–441, 1987. A highly critical review of this line of research can be found in M. Stein et al., "Depression, the Immune System, and Health and Illness," *Arch Gen Psychiat 48:*171–177, 1991. The author maintains that it is premature to claim a connection between depression and disturbed immunity.
5. M. E. P. Seligman, *Helplessness: On Depression, Development, and Death,* San Francisco: W. H. Freeman, 1975.
6. The topic of the health consequences of partner loss has been reviewed by Wolfgang and Margaret Stroebe, *Bereavement and Health,* Cambridge, England: Cambridge Press, 1987. The role of social factors in illness-sparing is brilliantly reviewed by John Cassel, "The Contribution of the Social Environment to Host Resistance," *Am J Epidemiology 101:*107–123, 1976.
7. Weiner, op. cit.
8. The most convincing evidence for anxiety and depressive disorders sharing a common substrate can be found in J. I. Hudson and H. G. Pope, Jr., "Affective Spectrum Dis-

order: Does Antidepressant Response Identify a Family of Disorders with a Common Pathophysiology?" *Am J Psychiatry 147*:552–564, 1990. Early studies that established the connection between anxiety and depressive disorders are as follows: M. Roth et al., "Studies in the Classification of Affective Disorder: I. The Relationship between Anxiety States and Depressive Illness," *Brit J Psychiat 121*:147–161, 1972; C. Zitrin et al., "Treatment of Phobia I. Comparison of Imipramine Hydrochloride and Placebo," *Arch Gen Psychiat 40*:125–138, 1983; M. Roth and C. Q. Mountjoy, "The Distinction between Anxiety States and Depressive Disorders," in E. S. Paykel, ed., *Handbook of Affective Disorders*, New York: Guilford Press, 1982, pp. 70–92.

9. The evidence that eating disorders have a depressive substrate, in spite of the authors' bent toward other explanations, is found in W. J. Swift et al., "The Relationship between Affective Disorder and Eating Disorders: A Review of the Literature," *Am J Psychiatry 143*:290–299, 1986. Also see Hudson and Pope, op. cit., and D. P. Cantwell et al., "Anorexia Nervosa: An Affective Disorder?" *Arch Gen Psychiatry 34*:1087–1093, 1977.

   The evidence is much spottier for post-traumatic stress disorder. For representative studies, see S. Falcon et al., "Tricyclics: Possible Treatment for Post-Traumatic Stress Disorder," *J Clin Psychiatry 46*:385–389, 1985; and G. L. Hogben and R. B. Cornfeld, "Treatment of Traumatic War Neuroses with Phenelzine," *Arch Gen Psychiatry 38*:440–445, 1981.

10. S. Lesse, "Hypochondriasis and Psychosomatic Disorders Masking Depression," *Am J Psychotherapy 21*:607, 1967; S. Lesse, "The Masked Depression Syndrome—Results of Seventeen-Year Clinical Study," *Am J Psychotherapy 37*:456–475, 1983.

    Recent studies of psychosomatically masked depression have concentrated on chronic pain syndromes. See D. Blumer, "Chronic Pain as a Variant of Depressive Disease," *J Nerv Mental Disease 170*: 381–401, 1982; Also D. Blumer and M. Heilbronn, "Antidepressant Treatment for Chronic Pain," *Psychiatric Annals 14*:796–800, 1984.

11. Winokur did the original research establishing the connection between alcoholism and depression. See G. Winokur et al., "Depressive Disease: A Genetic Study," *Arch Gen Psychiatry 24*:135–144, 1971; idem, "Alcoholism: III. Diagnosis and Familial Psychiatric Illness in 259 Alcoholic Probands," *Arch Gen Psychiatry 23*:104–111, 1970. Further research support can be found in P. Loosen et al., "Thyrotropin Releasing Hormone (TRH) in Abstinent Alcoholic Men," *Am J Psychiatry 140*:1145–1149, 1983. In a major review article, Schuckit draws together the evidence of a close connection between alcoholism and depression but then takes great pains to argue that they are separate disorders; see M. A. Schuckit, "Genetic and Clinical Implications of Alcoholism and Affective Disorder," *Am J Psychiatry 143*:140–147, 1986. From the biomedical perspective, all clinically distinguishable syndromes are presumed to have distinct biological profiles and therefore to be separate disorders. But this need not be so from the other perspectives making up the bio-existential hierarchy. For example, from the psychodynamic perspective, alcoholism is a specific, defensively elaborated form of depression or anxiety.

    For the relationship between depression and narcotics addiction, see B. J. Rounsaville et al., "Diagnosis and Symptoms of Depression in Opiate Addicts," *Arch Gen Psychiatry 39*:151–156, 1982; H. D. Kleber et al., "Imipramine Treatment for Depression in Addicts," *Arch Gen Psychiatry 40*:649–653, 1983.

    For the relationship between mood disorder and compulsive gambling, see R. A. McCormick, "Affective Disorders among Pathological Gamblers Seeking Treatment," *Am J Psychiatry 141*:215–218, 1984. The association between affective illness and compulsive exercising, shopping, telephoning, and sexual cruising, although frequently observed and often successfully treated clinically, has not been established in controlled studies.

For the relationship between affective, borderline, hysterical, conduct, and other acting-out personality disorders, the following studies are relevant: B. J. Carroll, "Neuroendocrine Evaluation of Depression in Borderline Patients," *Psychiat Clin N Amer 4*:89–99, 1981; H. S. Akiskal, "Borderline: An Adjective in Search of a Noun," *J Clin Psychiatry 46*:41–48, 1985; G. A. Carlson and D. P. Cantwell, "Unmasking Masked Depression in Children and Adolescents," *Am J Psychiatry 137*:445–449, 1980.

12. An excellent review article is G. Rodin and K. Voshart, "Depression in the Medically Ill," *Am J Psychiatry 143*:696–705, 1986.
13. For the notion of depression as a psychobiological final common pathway, see H. S. Akiskal and W. T. McKinney, "Overview of Recent Research in Depression," *Arch Gen Psychiatry 32*:285–305, 1975.
14. J. M. Mossey, K. Knott, and R. Craik, "The Effects of Persistent Depressive Symptoms on Hip Fracture Recovery," *J Gerontology: Medical Sciences 45*:M163–168, 1990.
15. J. R. Lipsey, R. G. Robinson, G. D. Pearlson, et al., "Nontriptyline Treatment of Post-Stroke Depression: A Double Blind Study," *Lancet 1*:297–300, 1984; W. Katon and M. Raskind, "Treatment of Depression in the Medically Ill Elderly with Methylphenidate," *Am J Psychiatry 137*:963–965, 1980.
16. T. H. Holmes and R. H. Rahe, "The Social Readjustment Scale," *J Psychosom Res 11*:213–218, 1967; also T. H. Holmes and M. Masuda, "Life Change and Illness Susceptibility," in B. S. Dohrenwend and B. P. Dohrenwend, eds., *Stressful Life Events*, New York: John Wiley, 1974. Paykel's work on early losses and subsequent depression is reviewed in E. S. Paykel, "Life Events and Early Environment," in E. S. Paykel, ed., *Handbook of Affective Disorders*, New York: Guilford Press, 1982.
17. G. L. Engel, "A Life Setting Conducive to Illness: The Giving Up, Given Up Complex," *Arch Internal Med 69*:293–300, 1968.
18. A. H. Schmale, Jr., "Relation of Separation and Depression to Disease: I. A Report on a Hospitalized Medical Population," *Psychosom Med 39*:344–357, 1977.
19. See note 3.
20. See note 12.
21. This study was originally done by M. Young, B. Benjamin, and C. Wallis, "Mortality of Widowers," *Lancet 2*:254–6, 1963; and followed up by Parkes et al., "Broken Heart: A Statistical Study of Increased Mortality among Widowers," *Brit Med J 1*:740–743, 1969.
22. K. Kahlbaum, *Catatonia*, Baltimore: Johns Hopkins Press, 1973; A. Meyer, *The Collected papers of Adolph Meyer, Volume 2: Psychiatry*, Baltimore: Johns Hopkins Press, 1951, pp. 444–445.
23. M. Day and E. V. Semrad, "Schizophrenic Reactions," in A. M. Nicholi, Jr., ed., *Harvard Guide to Modern Psychiatry*, Cambridge, MA: Harvard University Press, 1978.
24. S. S. Roth, "The Seemingly Ubiquitous Depression Following Acute Schizophrenic Episodes: A Neglected Area of Clinical Discussion," *Am J Psychiatry 127*:51–58, 1974; T. H. McGlashan and W. T. Carpenter, "Postpsychotic Depression in Schizophrenia," *Arch Gen Psychiatry 33*:231–239, 1976.
25. W. E. Broadhead et al., "The Epidemiological Evidence for a Relationship between Social Support and Health," *Am J Epidemiology 117*:521–537, 1983.
26. N. C. Andreasen, "Creativity and Mental Illness: Prevalence Rates in Writers and Their First Degree Relatives," *Am J Psychiatry 144*:1288–1292, 1987. Also see R. A. Woodruff et al., "Manic-Depressive Illness and Social Achievement," *Acta Psychiatr Scand 47*:237–249, 1971.

27. The work of Ruth Richards and Dennis Kinney suggests that it is not the full-blown affective syndromes but the minor variants, such as found in the relatives of manic-depressives, that lead to creative achievement. See article on creativity in the *New York Times*, Sept 13, 1988, page C1.
28. S. Freud, "On the Grounds for Detaching a Particular Syndrome from Neurasthenia under the Description of 'Anxiety Neurosis,'" in *The Standard Edition of the Complete Psychological Works of Sigmund Freud, Vol. 3,* London: Hogarth Press, 1962.

CHAPTER 8

The Dynamics of Drug Therapy

It is commonly assumed that whether or not medications are effective is largely a matter of their pharmacological properties: how well they reach the site of disorder, and how proficient they are at correcting the biological abnormalities present there. When antibiotics cure cases of pneumonia and antidepressants reverse the symptoms of depression while exacerbating those of mania, the common assumptions seem to hold up. The medicines work or fail to work because of their specific biological interactions.

This neat, simple way of looking at things begins to falter, however, in the presence of the placebo effect, which refers to the influence of psychological and existential factors on drug response. Because of suggestibility and positive expectations, some medications give a measure of relief that goes beyond their purely pharmacological potency. As a result of faith in the healer or his or her methods, even a chemically inert or irrelevant substance can lead to full symptomatic recovery. These phenomena allow quacks to feast on the gullibility of the desperate and competent practitioners to achieve results that are less the fruits of medical than of psychological influence.

The placebo effect also makes it extremely difficult to *prove* whether or not a medication is physiologically effective. Very sophisticated research designs, such as controlled, double-blind crossover studies, have to be carried out to come up with credible results. What complicates matters even further is the existence of *negative* placebo reactions. Equally pervasive as positive placebo responses (the nonbiological favorable reactions to medication) are nonspecific harmful effects that also derive from psychosocial and existential factors. As the reader has seen previously, patients often manifest serious resistance to being helped by drugs. They may refuse to take them at all, or if they do try, they may work against allowing or recognizing their positive effects. They may complain bitterly of minor side effects or unlikely complications that preclude continuing treatment, sometimes even in the face of significant benefits.

I have given several examples of negative placebo phenomena and their modification. In the case of Howard (recounted in Chapter 4), 6 years of psychotherapy elapsed before his resistance to taking antidepressants, particularly his intolerance of minor side effects, was overcome. To achieve this result, I had to devise strategies for inducing him to let me feed him. This orally defiant young man, who had developed an eating disorder at age 5, would never let anyone else nourish him prior to psychotherapy. He had to be convinced that it was safe to let both Beth and myself do it before he could utilize an antidepressant as a source of strength rather than weakness.

Similarly, Henry, discussed in Chapter 6, had run through a string of physicians and medications over many years' time before he allowed me to medicate away his gastrointestinal symptoms. I had already failed to help him with several antidepressants, the general class of drugs that eventually proved effective. In the meanwhile, he made it clear that he regarded doctors and medicines as noxious agents and that, by defeating them, he was triumphing over the poisonous treatment accorded him by his wife and mother. To overcome his resistance, I had to convince him that my prescription of a medicine was a caring rather than a poisonous act. I did this in several ways: by writing him a warm letter asking him to return to treatment, by giving credence and support to his resistance, and by definitively (after some false starts) taking his side in his struggle with his wife.

I would like to accomplish two tasks in this chapter: first, to review the various bio-existential components of the medication response; and second, to categorize and provide examples of negative placebo effects and the means of overcoming them. The major studies of placebo effects were carried out by Jerome Frank,[1] whose definition of psychotherapy was described in Chapter 2, and Arthur Shapiro,[2] to whose work I am particularly indebted in the following discussion.

THE ELEMENTS OF THE MEDICATION RESPONSE

All accounts of medication effects must begin with the biomedical foundation—the purely pharmacological aspects of psychoactive drug response. Currently, psychiatrists utilize five main types of agents: (a) *antidepressants,* which diminish the mood, sleep, eating, energy, and pleasure disturbances of depressive disorders; the panic, phobic, and obsessive-compulsive symptoms of anxiety disorders; and the physical symptoms of psychosomatic conditions, presumably by affecting serotonin, norepinephrine, and related neurotransmitters and their receptors in the limbic system of the brain; (b) *mood stabilizers* (e.g., lithium, carbamazepine, clonazepam, and valproic acid), which have antimanic, antidepressant, and anticonvulsant properties, operating through second-messenger systems, sodium and calcium channels, and GABA transmission; (c) *antipsychotics* or *neuroleptics,* which diminish delusions, hallucinations, and disorganized, withdrawn, or bizarre behaviors (including their subpsychotic forms), presumably by affecting dopamine transmission in the central nervous system; (d) *anxiolytic-sedatives,* which diminish symptoms of panic, hyperventilation, palpitations, muscle tension, insomnia, anticipatory anxiety, and phobic fears by affecting the GABA system; and (e) *psychostimulants,* which diminish the symptoms of attention deficit disorder by mechanisms that are poorly understood.[3]

What *is* understood is that these various agents, when prescribed in the right amounts for the right symptoms, will have significant benefits in 60% to 70% of cases, largely on the basis of their biomedical properties but assisted by the placebo effect. Of the nonresponders, some no doubt have biologically variant or concurrent disorders that require alternative agents, either already available or yet to be developed. While every effort continues to be made to find effective alternative regimes, the most fruitful clinical strategy is to regard the residual nonresponders as having negative placebo reactions—absent or adverse effects mainly on psychosocial and existential grounds—and to work at overcoming these. To be sure, there is a large area of overlap here. A hypersensitive paranoid patient who reacts violently to the minor sedative effects of a neuroleptic agent might become less resistant to a more effective, less sedating agent, one that chemically reduces the paranoid fear of psychoactive medication more definitively. Quite clearly, then, even resistance has both biological and psychological roots. In understanding drug response, the two factors can never be strictly separated.

The most basic psychological aspects of medication response are encompassed by the learning theory framework. From this perspective, both positive and negative drug effects derive from the past conditioning of patients and their current perceptions of what is expected of them. Highly traumatic or highly favorable past experiences with doctors and their drugs and mothers and their milk surely influence, by the mechanisms of classical conditioning, how individuals react to proffered medication in the present. Patients are also sensitive to subtle and not-so-subtle operant cues: what the prestigious drug prescriber expects in the way of a response, what the rewards (approval alone can make a powerful appeal) will be for meeting these expectations, and what the penalties will be for not doing so.

Thus, from the learning theory perspective, physicians, therapists, and experimenters to a significant degree shape the drug responses of subjects by their communicated interests, their capacity to suggest and persuade, and their stimulus value in evoking the positive and negative conditions of past treatments. As a consequence, valued therapists who consciously or unconsciously disapprove of their clients' taking psychoactive medications tend to reinforce and amplify side effects and minimize positive benefits, with the result that the outcome is perceived as unsatisfactory. Conversely, enthusiastic patients and therapists tend to amplify positive effects and to convince themselves of a favorable outcome, at least temporarily.

From the psychodynamic perspective, the patient-therapist drug interaction is permeated with transference phenomena in general and with developmental factors in particular. It may, moreover, be entirely sabotaged by dissociated subpersonalities that try to veto all effective treatment methods. In this model, the patient displaces onto the drug prescriber attitudes toward parental figures from childhood. If these are positive, the placebo effects will be favorable. If the patient's internal saboteur mobilizes negative transference, then placebo effects will be mostly negative. As the readers will soon see, the type of placebo response can be more specifically related to the individual's psychosexual and psychosocial stage of development.

The individual is also subjected to enormous social pressure either to take psychoactive medication and experience benefits or to refuse to cooperate with recommended drug regimes. As already implied, the social prestige of the physician is a major factor here, and the esteem of peers and society at large can make the difference as to whether medication is effective or not. Thus, patients undergoing group therapy have a much better chance of deriving benefits if fellow members have had good results and are persuasive about the positive benefits and the harmlessness of side effects. Conversely, other groups (e.g., Alcoholics Anonymous) tend to dissuade patients from trying therapeutic drugs, which they characterize in terms little different from those referring to narcotics.

From the existential vantage point, response to psychoactive drugs is a matter of beliefs and values. Certainly a strong case can be made for trying to surmount mental problems by insight and determination alone, without taking the apparently "easy" route of swallowing chemicals. Such an approach places high value on discipline and active striving, a strengthening of the will that refuses to bow to ordinary pain and adversity. From such a vantage point, having to take a tranquilizer or an antidepressant is experienced as a moral defeat, a sign of weakness of character, or a tendency toward "psychotropic hedonism."[4] An alternative value position regards mental symptoms as in part the manifestations of deficiency diseases, on the order of diabetes. Not to take an antidepressant in the face of the correct diagnosis would be as self-destructive and inconsiderate of loved ones as not taking insulin for high blood sugar. The common thread running through these considerations is the power of beliefs to determine drug response. A belief in the essential goodness or evil, or potency or impotency, of modern medical science has everything to do with how drug therapy is perceived and takes effect. Just as important is the patient's faith in physicians and therapists and their essential power, beneficence, and competence.

The main point is that any one of these factors—faith, transference, social pressure, or operant and classical conditioning—can operate with enough power in the individual case to override the purely pharmacological effects of a medication. An effective drug can be immeasurably enhanced or fatally undermined by these nonbiological forces, so that a skillful marshaling of them for therapeutic objectives (i.e., the ability to enhance the positive placebo effect) becomes one of the most important skills of the modern, drug-prescribing bio-existential therapist. Yet it remains one of the most neglected areas of conventional mental treatment and training.

SPECIFIC FORMS OF RESISTANCE TO MEDICATION

Resistance to taking one's medication, no less than resistance to looking at one's motivation, can strike a decisive blow against one's success not only in therapy but in life in general. The salesman who has been laid off repeatedly for angry manic outbursts effectively ruins both his career and his marriage by adamantly refusing, for reasons he cannot adequately explain, to take the lithium preparation that has in the past prevented his self-destructive behavior. The parents of a bulimic adolescent girl sentence her to years of misery by forbidding her to take the antidepressant that controls her binge eating. Even when she resolves to continue it without their permission, she involuntarily throws up all the pills. By declining to take small doses of a neuroleptic that he says gives him body odor, a paranoid patient is consigned to living in a world full of hateful enemies who rob him of all satisfaction.

Yet these same patients often have less trouble taking such nonpsychoactive substances as vitamins, antibiotics, or medicinals acquired from nonphysicians. Why the special resistance to "mind-altering" agents and the prescriptions of doctors? To answer these questions, we have to look more closely at the dynamics of taking psychoactive drugs. Up to now, I have referred to all cases of resistance under the rubric of negative placebo reaction. To classify them more precisely, we need to look at the impact of psychosocial development on drug taking. Whereas normal development leads to straightforward cooperation tempered by healthy skepticism in following drug regimens, arrests in the maturational process—in traversing the oral, anal, and genital stages—can generate serious disturbances in the sense of trust, autonomy, and integrity necessary to deriving optimal benefits from drug therapy.

Medication and Mistrust

Taking a powerful psychoactive medication from a physician immediately raises the question of trust. Can the doctor be relied upon to provide safe and effective care? Those who have been the victims of serious mistreatment and failures of empathy by parents and caregivers in the past do not readily assume that they are in reliable hands. Based on past experience, they doubt the competence or good intentions of psychiatrists and the beneficial nature of what they have to offer. Particularly if early mothering has been psychotically abusive or otherwise so frustrating as to arouse murderous rage, then all future attempts to provide care may be experienced as potentially lethal. This is especially the case for powerful medications that can in fact have harmful side effects. At the very least, a fear of being poisoned or intoxicated can be stirred up.

For example, Carla, a 50-year-old professional woman, was subjected to constant abuse as a child by her psychotic mother. She was frequently harangued, disowned for minor transgressions, and advised not to socialize with neighborhood children or take the advice of teachers. Now depressed as an adult, she found it extremely difficult to take medication for her symptoms. She called repeatedly to be reassured that desipramine had no dangerous effects. Anxieties apparently allayed, she then discovered that she could not swallow the tablets; they got stuck in the back of her throat. Advised to take them dissolved in orange juice, she became panic stricken, certain that she would die if she swallowed the liquid.

Two weeks of almost continual reassurance were required before Carla was successful, and even then she initially had to ingest the desipramine in my presence. Once she was able to take it, however, she had no trouble letting it work or tolerating its side effects. She soon noted an improved sense of well-being and, most notably, a marked diminution in her indecisiveness and procrastination.

In retrospect, Carla realized that she regarded her mother as so injurious and hateful that from the age of 4 on, she began bathing and dressing herself, refusing all offers of her mother's care and taking every opportunity to dine with neighbors despite her mother's paranoid warnings about them. Because of the strengthening effects of the antidepressant she was able to reexperience the pain of her childhood and to see how fearful she had been of her mother's criticisms and interrogatations and how she had transferred these feelings to me and the concrete help I was offering her. The biological intervention led to new insights on the psychodynamic plane.

As the reader has seen in past clinical examples, particularly the case of Henry, other patients will take medication with little overt anxiety but then amplify ordinary side effects to the level of intolerable severity. Or they will go through the *Physicians' Desk Reference* with a fine-toothed comb and become convinced that all the rare adverse reactions listed are not only possible but probable. Generally, these are cases in which the fear of being poisoned is in large measure unconscious. While initially denying any concern over toxicity, many of these patients can be helped to uncover the underlying feelings and to resolve them. In all such cases, psychodynamic insight is of course helpful, but it needs to be given teeth by the behavioral techniques of repeated exposure to medication and the prevention of avoidance responses.

The other main manifestation of disturbance at the stage of oral trust-mistrust is the "addictive" reaction to offered medication. This usually takes two different forms: actual addictive behavior, or an irrational fear of becoming addicted. The first phenomenon occurs in patients with addictive personalities, who respond to all medications as if they were "hooked" on them. Given a nonaddictive antidepressant, these voraciously needy individuals will become frantic about their dosage schedule, worrying that they have been given too much or too little. They often get the pharmacy to call to renew prescriptions long before they have run out. They constantly change their dose without consulting their psychiatrist or therapist, thereby getting into problems of over- or undermedication. Their preoccupation with and excessive reliance on chemical agents typically comes at the expense of the repeated acts of will and the discipline that ensure psychological growth. Thus, they have to be helped gradually to change their focus and to overcome these bad habits of thought and behavior.

In the other form of the addictive response, patients will decline or resist taking medications because of a fear of becoming dependent on them. Because they do not usually have addictive personalities, the fear can usually be regarded as irrational and therefore vigorously combatted. To begin with, what is needed are educational sessions devoted to the facts of addiction and how most psychoactive drugs fail to induce the craving, tolerance, and withdrawal symptoms characteristic of chemical dependency. Even in the case of the benzodiazepines, which can cause dependency, an exploration of the warning signs and a willingness to change to longer-acting agents usually makes it possible to vouch for the relative safety of this class of drugs.

Of course, rational discussions are not always sufficient, especially when behavior has deep emotional roots. For example, one patient who had a very favorable response to fluoxetine periodically stopped taking it, always with a disastrous return of low spirits, agitation, and palpitations. On each occasion, her fears of becoming too dependent on the medication overwhelmed her. She asked me each time, "Are you sure I'm not addicted? Isn't this just a crutch? What happens if I lose my suitcase on a trip and can't get a new prescription?" Each time I went over the familiar ground, explaining how some medications like insulin make good on a biological deficiency but, unlike cocaine and other narcotics, do not stimulate uncontrollable drug seeking or necessitate ever-higher doses. Although convinced anew each time, she continued to repeat the cycle for 3 years before she was finally able to stay on the medication without interruption. Significantly, she was hardly bothered by the negative publicity concerning fluoxetine's potentially dangerous side effects. Fear of toxicity was simply not her issue.

Medication and Autonomy

Excessively harsh or rigid training that violates the child's basic sense of autonomy will often result in adult patients who approach taking medication in either an overly compliant or oppositional manner. In the first instance, seemingly intelligent individuals will blindly follow prescriptions that are clearly harmful. For example, a highly compulsive university professor with crippling anxiety came for an evaluation on seven different medications (Elavil, Valium, Placidyl, Seconal, Stelazine, and vitamin B_{12}), mostly in subtherapeutic dosages but enough all together to cause crippling sedation. Only because of his wife's nagging did he come for another opinion. He had never before questioned the authority or effectiveness of any of his physicians.

By contrast, some patients get into a power struggle over even the most straightforward prescribing issues. Virtually all treatment suggestions, and particularly those involving medication, arouse these patients' fears of being externally controlled. This phenomenon is often connected in the patient's mind with the fear of being subjected to hypnosis, brainwashing, or indoctrination, all of which involve falling under the influence of an alien, potentially harmful outside force. One of the main dangers of such suspicious, defiant reactions is that the patients will validate their fears by provoking a retaliatory response in the physician. Needless to say, success in working with this kind of patient involves learning not to rise to the bait. Instead, the most nondirective stance possible must be adopted: explaining the pros and cons of the various options, clearly leaving the final choices about taking medication to the patient, and discussing the limited potency of biological agents, compared to the power of the will, in promoting or resisting changes. In such cases we see most clearly the importance of presenting psychoactive agents as mere adjuncts to therapy—aids to the patient's own efforts to get better, certainly not the most important factor.

Medication and Integrity

Another major category of resistance to taking psychoactive medications concerns the fear of losing psychobiological integrity. Patients who have had difficulties in traversing the genital stage may respond to recommended drugs with severe "castration anxiety." Taking the medication stirs up feelings of being physically defective, weakened, violated, or penetrated. The wholeness of the organism feels assaulted, not only by the act of taking medicine but sometimes even by being advised to do so. Such patients are apt to leave the recommending therapist's office with great resentment, as if the suggestion inflicted a severe injury on their masculine or feminine competence. When advised to go on an antidepressant, a law enforcement officer asked me if I was trying to turn him into a woman!

A more complex example: Ruth, a 35-year-old divorced law student, was referred for evaluation of depressive symptoms and unsuccessful relationships with men. The referring therapist was aware that taking medicine was a loaded issue for Ruth, but only cursorily prepared her for the consultation. Coming to see a male psychiatrist with the power to make a medical diagnosis and prescribe medical treatment was such a frightening prospect for Ruth that she got lost on the way to my office and arrived 20 minutes late. Making haste rather than good sense, I rushed through the evaluation in the half hour that remained. Eliciting clear vegetative signs of a long-standing biological depression, I felt very confident that the shortened session had not materially affected the thoroughness and quality of my evaluation and confidently recommended a trial of antidepressant medication. I also told her I would supplement our time together by a series of phone contacts to evaluate her drug response.

Ruth agreed to try the medicine and check in by phone, but she showed some discomfort as she wrote out the check for my consultation fee. Although she did not vent her feelings to me, she told her therapist that she had been "shafted" and "ripped off," that I had pushed medicines on her without having time to get to know her and that I had overcharged her. She felt "fucked," as she always was by men. When this information came back to me, I offered Ruth a free makeup session. She accepted but spent the whole time telling me how badly treated she had felt, without being consoled by my efforts at conciliation. Subsequently, I alerted her therapist to the presence of powerful resistances to taking medication and suggested that the same forces—mainly, a fear of being penetrated—might be operating in her love life. Soon thereafter, the patient stopped checking in with me and discontinued her antidepressant.

A year later, after she had worked in therapy on her sense of violation by me, characteristic of her relationships with the significant males in her life, Ruth returned for another, more successful trial of drug therapy. With much coaxing and soothing she was able to take small amounts of trifluoperazine, which markedly reduced her paranoid suspiciousness, and then fluoxetine for her depressive symptoms. Moreover, she agreed to see me monthly, both for medication checks and to learn to have a comfortable relationship with a man whom she regarded as powerful. Gradually, this paid off in her ability to have a sustained, intimate relationship, and eventually to get married.

Medication and Forced Maturation

One final source of resistance to taking psychoactive medication is the fear of psychological growth. Becoming energized by antidepressants or cognitively focused by neuroleptics may put enormous pressures on the patient to move forward in life, particularly to give up destructive, infantile relationships and activities. But these unhealthy attachments, sometimes involving long-standing bad marriages, passive habits, and frustrating jobs, may be too strong to relinquish easily. For example, once she went on lithium, Beth realized that her relationship to her first boyfriend was appallingly childish. But even though she resolved to give him up, she needed a great deal of social pressure and support before she could do it.

Many patients are simply unable to make such changes, particularly when they have been locked into an unsuitable marriage or career for many years. For example, when Edie, a housewife in her mid-30s, became undepressed on fluoxetine, she could no longer deny that her husband was not holding up his end of the relationship and that she deserved better: someone who showed up regularly at work and who earned a decent living and had time for her and the children. Despite her urging he refused to go for help. Instead of leaving him, however, she stopped her fluoxetine and sank back into the life of quiet misery that she knew so well. In another case, the patient's husband objected to her going on psychoactive medicine because he was accustomed to talking over her many problems with her every day after work. He was quite frank in admitting that if her symptoms remitted on medication, he would lose one of the main sources of pleasure in their relationship. Instead of being repelled by such exploitation, the patient decided to put off a decision on medication—a delay that is now approaching 3 years in duration.

Similarly, some patients go off their lithium because they miss the highs they are accustomed to; on the medication, the mess they have made of their lives and the hard work needed to set things straight cannot so readily be obscured in the fog of grandiose rationalizations. In contrast, a professional writer threw her antidepressant away because it banished the feeling of *weltschmerz* out of which she wrote all her best pieces. A well paid executive hated his job but was too depressed and cognitively unfocused to know why. On 75 mg a day of nortriptyline he saw altogether too well that his boss was stealing from the company and had him involved in the deception. But where was he going to get another job that paid so well? Though at first feeling improved on the medication, he soon found himself sleepy at work and needing to take frequent naps, which he now blamed on the nortriptyline despite my best interpretive efforts. Once he decided to stop it, he felt more alert and better able to forget his complaints about the job.

Some patients are clearly not able to handle comfortably the forward developmental pressure generated by good drug therapy. Whenever possible, they should be helped to see the source of their discomfort, hopefully as a first step to overcoming the resistance to growth. But in some cases the cost of change is too great, even dangerous to psychic balance.

The prospect of growth stirs up intolerable anxieties and may even threaten an uncontrolled regression.

PRINCIPLES OF PRESCRIBING

I have explored some of the main resistances, or negative placebo factors, involved in psychoactive drug prescribing. Quite clearly, these have to be overcome if patients are to receive optimal multidimensional therapy. Some of the practical ways of achieving this goal have been touched on in the foregoing clinical examples. To amplify this prior discussion, I would suggest that the following procedures be followed once the correct diagnosis and drug selection have been made.

First, the patient's attitudes toward and history of psychoactive drug taking should be elicited. If there are no signs of serious resistances, then it is safe to move to the second step, which is to provide information as to the rationale for the recommended drug therapy, its mode of action, common side effects, rare dangers, and general safety. This information should be presented in a persuasive manner that elicits consent and cooperation yet informs the patient of the possible grounds for refusing. If serious biases and resistances are uncovered in the first step, then the therapist should move to the third step of providing both the scientific information and psychodynamic insights necessary to removing these barriers. If the patient agrees to take medication but gives evidence of residual resistance by exaggerating side effects, then the psychiatrist should adopt the behavioral strategy of repeated exposure to varying doses and agents and firm pressure to resist avoidance responses.

If, after being provided with information and analysis of resistance, the patient still declines to try medication in the face of strong indications, then a holographic intervention might be devised: a behavioral analogue of drug taking that, if the patient carries it out, overcomes the whole psychological basis of the negative placebo reaction. As the reader saw in the case of Howard, this involved first getting him (by a complicated maneuver) to accept the gift of a recording from me. In other patients, it may involve getting them to try recommended restaurants and even special dishes as a prelude to following recommendations about medication.

Yet in our zeal to overcome resistances, we must not fail to acknowledge the very real opposite danger of overprescribing. This is a particular danger of the biomedical emphasis of the bio-existential approach, which in postulating a depressive substrate to most mental and psychosomatic disorders encourages widespread pharmacological interventions.

To avoid both under- and overprescribing and to ensure careful follow-up of drug therapy, I have found the following maxims to be extremely useful in improving the results of treatment.

Do not rush into prescribing. Of course, some patients, because of severe suffering or danger, need to be medicated right away. But for the majority there is no great urgency in giving or sending the patient for medication, and there are many advantages to holding off until a strong therapeutic alliance has been formed. This involves not only generating a mutual feeling of trust and respect but a knowledge of the patient's attitudes toward receiving help in general and medication in particular. Past drug history, including substance abuse, must be carefully evaluated. Any record of misuse or untoward effects, as well as of prudent usage and strong benefits, must be carefully searched out. In such matters, the past is always the best predictor of the future. From the therapy perspective, the aim is to get patients to enhance positive placebo effects and diminish negative ones. Making certain that the offering of medication is received as a nurturing, caring gift rather than a controlling, poisonous attack can sometimes take months to years of preparation. The improved results are worth the effort.

Medication must be carefully monitored, and in a way that stimulates the patient's initiative. The twin dangers of drug therapy—losing control over powerful medication effects, and instilling passive-dependent attitudes in patients—make it important that drug therapy be carefully supervised. The best modes of supervision are those that counteract the passivity-inducing effects of merely taking pills and counting on their help; rather, active participation has to be sought. The best methods for accomplishing this are to have patients keep written records of their responses and call in regularly to report these effects so that modifications in regimens can be made promptly. By insisting that clients make these calls punctually and convey information concisely and thoroughly, both active collaboration and heightened cognitive organization are encouraged. At the same time, patients are trained to become more sensitively attuned to their own feelings and attitudes. As the reader will see in the next chapter, however, telephone reporting—which involves a bending of traditional therapy rules—is not without danger and therefore has to be judiciously prescribed.

Medication dosage should be lowered as soon as feasible. As mentioned earlier, the potency of psychoactive medications should not be oversold. Instead, their effects should generally be characterized as providing modest and partial solutions to mental problems. In some cases, they may be used only to provide a "reference experience," that is, to give the first experience of a desired mental state that can subsequently be reclaimed psychologically without further reliance on chemical agents. In other words, these therapeutic drug "flashbacks" can often be invoked at will, lessening or obviating the need for current drug taking.

Again, in fostering attitudes of active utilization rather than passive compliance, patients are encouraged to get by with less or no medication after their clinical condition has stabilized for several months. Then, gradual tapering while looking for recurrent symptoms is attempted. Of course, clinical worsening dictates that doses be promptly increased again but then, with prolonged stability or increased side effects, reduced slowly once more to the point just short of symptom recurrence.

While this is going on, therapy is directed toward retaining drug benefits by active mental and physical striving. All the therapeutic approaches to mood and thought disorders encompassed by the other four bio-existential traditions are constantly and energetically applied to make the patient less exclusively reliant on biomedical agents and more on his or her own psychological and spiritual resources. For example, as part of their behavioral and cognitive therapy treatment, patients on antidepressants and mood stabilizers should when possible be involved in vigorous physical fitness and assertiveness training programs. And those on neuroleptics for thought disorder should carry out programs for instituting tighter structure, order, and boundaries in their lives. Resistances to such vital activities are routinely confronted, and all the psychosocial techniques deployed to overcome them.

Thus, medication is presented as a possibly temporary internal splint that provides the support for patients to repair and strengthen their mental functioning. Once the needed psychological and existential growth has been accomplished, then some or all of the splint can be removed. With neurotic and mild borderline levels of mood and thought disorder, a properly conducted psychotherapy should eventually permit the full removal of the biological splint. In more severe borderline and psychotic conditions, however, some or all of it may have to be retained indefinitely or, in special circumstances, temporarily stopped and reinstituted at periodic intervals. Yet we must not forget that for some patients, symptom production is under such strong biological pressure that drug therapy has to be continued at full therapeutic levels indefinitely.

Drug therapy must be tailored to personality patterns and prognosis. The presentation of psychoactive drugs should be varied according to the patterns and goals of individual patients. Those who have a history of profiting from drug therapy and utilizing it to facilitate personal growth can be managed in a much more straightforward fashion than those who have had mostly unsuccessful trials in the past. The latter must be carefully evaluated to determine whether the problem is attitudinal or biological (i.e., attributable to resistance or a suboptimal drug regimen). In some cases, it becomes painfully obvious that no psychoactive medication is likely to afford relief, at least in the current state of our knowledge.

As has been discussed, some alcoholic, drug-abusing, passive-dependent, and eating-disordered patients tend to utilize the medications like addictive substances, taking too little or too much of them and developing magical expectations about their effects. In such cases, drugs must be prescribed very sparingly and for very limited goals. Their potential benefits may have to be played down while possible side effects are emphasized. In contrast, other patients, particularly obsessive-compulsives who become paralyzed by indecision and doubt, may have to be firmly directed to take medication without too many disclaimers or expressed concerns about adverse effects.

The referral process, vulnerable to the same resistances as found in individual patients, has to be carefully managed. The increasing reliance on psychoactive medication, and therefore the increased need for collaboration between medical and nonmedical therapists, has generated additional sources of negative placebo reactions. In making referrals for biomedical evaluation, therapists can contaminate their clients' responses to medication by adding their own, often unconscious, fears and biases to the situation. If both therapist and client have fears of being poisoned, controlled, or violated and these fears interact synergistically, then the likelihood of adverse reactions and frank failures becomes a virtual certainty. For example, in the case of Ruth discussed earlier, the referring therapist did not adequately prepare the patient for the consultation. She did not inform Ruth of my fee, discuss my likely diagnoses and recommendations, or warn the patient about my decisiveness in making them, all of which she knew from past experience. Nor did she fully explore the patient's fears of coming for the evaluation. Sometimes these are so strong that they can be mitigated only by having the therapist physically accompany the client to the psychiatric consultation.

In this case, as became apparent from our subsequent discussions, the therapist had developed renewed doubts about the safety of antidepressants and had lingering fears about their capacity to exert undue behavioral control. These unaddressed concerns interfered with her giving the referral the careful attention it required. Yet in view of the intensity of Ruth's neurotic conflicts, there is some doubt that all difficulties could have been avoided even with the best referral.

Giving and receiving psychoactive medication is both biological and psychosocial intercourse. What this means is that prescribing should always be regarded as a multilevel, penetrating interaction. It is never just a medical event but always has psychosocial and existential parameters. To be sure, because there are important individual biological differences that may account for poor drug response, psychiatrists and therapists have to be prepared to try multiple agents to find optimally effective ones. But at a certain point, persistent treatment failures have to be looked at as failures in intercourse caused by the usual inhibitions that produce symptoms of "impotence" and "frigidity": performance and castration anxiety, oral rage, incest taboo, fear of penetration, and loss of identity and independence. This means that special attention may have to be given to promote a positive response: Therapists may have to work hard to become better attuned to the patient's special needs, to provide the support and tenderness that enlists cooperation, and the caring firmness that curbs rebellion. Above all, patience and understanding will have to be shown in abundance.

If possible, do not represcribe medications that have failed in the past, even if the failure was the result of subsequently resolved resistances. As will become apparent from reviewing the cases of Henry and Howard, I carefully avoid demonstrating to patients that their own disowned feelings and attitudes were the cause of drug failures. By always moving on to new agents, I give them the "out" that lack of success was at least in part pharmacological. In the process, I avoid ramming the medications down the throat of the patient's unconscious (i.e., proving that the problem was psychological resistance), instead leaving open the possibility that the new medication is better suited biologically. Although this approach can result in a loss of potential scientific knowledge, it often compensates with a gain in clinical effect. As Schopenhauer first pointed out, the unconscious will does not always like to be made aware of its own workings. If its aims are unnecessarily exposed, it is apt sooner or later to retaliate by committing new acts of sabotage.

SUMMARY AND CONCLUSIONS

Taking psychoactive medications may stir up fears of being poisoned, addicted, controlled, castrated, or violated. In addition, it may put the patient under intense maturational pressure, calling for difficult renunciations of infantile attachments and pleasures. Unresolved conflicts of these issues may lead to blocks in accepting that medications are indicated or, more strikingly, in simply swallowing them, tolerating their side effects, and allowing them to exert their psychobiological benefits. A psychotherapeutic approach to such resistances—involving educational discussions and attention to operant and classical conditioning, conflict-anxiety, internal saboteurs, social pressure, and reigning values—is often highly effective in obtaining positive benefits in cases initially characterized by noncompliance or negative reactions.

In our zeal to overcome sources of resistance to psychoactive drug therapy, we must take steps to avoid overprescribing while fostering active mental striving. The importance of a strong therapeutic alliance and of careful monitoring and sensitive modification of drug regimens have been emphasized. Equally important, we have looked at the vulnerability of the referral process to antitherapeutic biases. Because the giving and receiving of medication is not just a medical transaction but a complex form of psychosocial intercourse, great attention must be paid to the usual ways of overcoming "impotence" and "frigidity." Thus, even though a judicious amount of psychological force may have to be deployed in prescribing agents that penetrate the inner space of clients, it should always be done in spirit of cooperation, never in a way that evokes feelings of undue control or violation.

NOTES

1. J. D. Frank, *Persuasion and Healing,* Baltimore: Johns Hopkins Press, 1961, pp. 65–74.
2. A. K. Shapiro and L. A. Morris, "The Placebo Effect In Medical and Psychological Therapies," in S. L. Garfield and A. E. Bergin, eds., *Handbook of Psychotherapy and Behavioral Change,* 2nd ed., New York: John Wiley, 1978, pp. 369–410.
3. See standard texts of psychoactive drug therapy; for example, G. W. Arana and S. E. Hyman, *Handbook of Psychiatric Drug Therapy,* 2nd. ed., Boston: Little, Brown, 1991.
4. For a fuller discussion of the value dimension of psychoactive drug therapy, see G. L. Klerman and G. Schecter, "Ethical Aspects of Drug Treatment," in S. Bloch and P. Chodoff, eds., *Psychiatric Ethics,* Oxford, England: Oxford University Press, 1961, pp. 117–130.

CHAPTER 9

Changing the Rules

Psychotherapy is "a circumscribed, structured series of contacts between a healer and a sufferer."[1] What this means is that it is a formal relationship bound by strictly formulated rules and obligations. Typically these dictate, for example, that the meetings take place at the therapist's office, not the patient's home, and that they occur for a defined duration and at a fixed frequency rather than according to the changing personal wishes of the participants (as is typical of ordinary friendships). Though adherence to such rules is designed to promote positive developmental changes, in some cases their observance is counterproductive because they lie too far outside the patient's capabilities or interests. In the image of the parable in Chapter 1, upholding them would be like insisting that the Vietnam veteran eat his birdseed in formal attire off Limoges china. In his delusion of being a bird, such a requirement would not only be offensive, but it would convince the soldier that he had fallen into enemy hands. A more effective approach, as the reader has seen, is to join patients where they are, to enter into their regressed-advanced worlds and then gradually lead them toward more socialized behavior.

Before exploring the indications for breaking the rules, however, I would first like to go over the main strictures of traditional psychotherapy to come to some understanding of their rationale. The following list starts with the most widely observed standard rules and proceeds to less commonly followed ones.

1. No sexual contact
2. Fee-for-service payment
3. Strict time and place boundaries
4. Focus on patient and away from therapist
5. Full disclosure from patient through free associations

6. Limited or no disclosure from therapist (i.e., blank-screen anonymity)
7. Therapist in charge of structure but nondirective of content
8. No socializing outside office
9. No value judgments about patient's social behavior (i.e., moral neutrality)
10. Verbal expression but no physical contact (e.g., no hugging, handshakes, hitting)
11. No communication with family, employers, friends (i.e., privacy and confidentiality)
12. No gifts
13. No use of first names
14. No avowed expectations of positive change in symptoms

As is well known, every one of these rules, including the first, is regularly violated by some therapists, while at least a few orthodox practitioners religiously follow them all. The vast majority, however, tend to follow the first few quite consistently and to make occasional or frequent exceptions to the rest. For example, in some cases it makes sense to attend the weddings and major celebrations of patients, not to mention family funerals. And there are circumstances in which shaking hands or patting backs contaminates therapy far less than failing to make physical contact. What is being implied is that although there are good reasons for obeying the standard rules, there are sometimes better reasons for setting them aside.

GENERAL RATIONALE OF THE RULES

The standard rules derive from the psychodynamic school, which is fundamentally an individual developmental therapy. Its main aim has always been to help neurotic patients move from an infantile, passive symbiotic consciousness to a mature, independent, reflective mode of awareness. Obeying the standard rules clearly has the effect of furthering this cause. The majority work to prevent patients from becoming dependently enmeshed with therapists, and instead foster individual insight, initiative, and responsibility. All the strictures involving fees, time and place, outside socializing, nondirectiveness, neutrality, privacy, and confidentiality have the effect of strengthening personal boundaries and diminishing the tendency of patients to fuse or become overly identified with therapists and significant others.

In addition, following the standard rules has the effect of evoking patients' immature, symptomatic behaviors so that they can be corrected. Expecting them to show up on time, leave promptly at the end of sessions, and pay bills regularly is bound to expose arrests in early psychosocial development. Such requirements evoke unresolved issues of dependency, retentiveness, disorganization, and grandiosity. The other procedures, such as encouraging fantasy while discouraging acting out, expose deficiencies in self-control and in mechanisms of delay and postponement. Finally, the emphasis on free-associated fantasy in the face of a cue-depriving, blank-screen therapist selectively lessens ego control, thereby evoking primary process thinking and previously unconscious primitive wishes and needs. This sets the stage for developing the transference neurosis: the reenactment with the therapist of problematic childhood relationships.

Moreover, the standard rules have a stabilizing effect on the therapeutic relationship. Observing them tends to provide ballast against the gushing resentments and attractions inevitably generated by working closely together. No matter how hurt, angry, or turned on, patients must still show up at the appointed time and place, ready to do the required work. And even if therapists become disgusted with patients' behavior and are tempted to reject them, they first analyze their own countertransference reactions and then refocus on the patient, asking "Why did you do that? Have you done it before? What was the outcome?" In the process they develop understanding and acceptance, to the immense benefit of the therapeutic process. Similarly, no matter how angry or enraptured clients become with therapists, they are taught to keep the focus on their own lives and the contribution to these attitudes of transferred, conditioned feelings from childhood.

Some of the rules also teach the essential ingredients of friendly and harmonious relationships. For example, by keeping the focus of attention on patients, therapists provide a good model of how to show interest in others. Similarly, the fee-for-service exchange potently teaches the necessity of reciprocal, fair exchanges in sustaining close relationships. It is hoped that as these ties become less formal and more intimate, the currency goes beyond monetary transactions to signs of caring and consideration, which are counted no less carefully (if less overtly) than exchanges of cash.

These are such intrinsically worthwhile aims and so workable in ordinary neurotic patients that it is sometimes difficult to see that they depend on preconditions that cannot usually be met in nonneurotic patients. But the very existence of the nonpsychodynamic schools of treatment speaks to this fact, for each of them violates the standard rules in order to make good on the deficits or special needs of those who are unsuited to individual psychodynamic therapy. We must now examine these justifications for breaking the rules.

RATIONALE FOR BREAKING THE RULES

It is commonly appreciated that the psychodynamic rules should not be enforced if patients are psychotic. "Parameters" have to be introduced in these cases (i.e., the rules have to be broken) because therapist anonymity, neutrality, and nondirectiveness tend to exacerbate psychotic symptoms. In fact, the very first patient I treated in my private practice, some 25 years ago, became ravingly paranoid as I sat behind her while she free-associated on the couch. She settled down only after I sat her up and persuaded her to take neuroleptic medication. In retrospect, I realized that I had missed the fact that she harbored delusional ideas. After treatment with trifluoperazine and enhanced structure and face-to-face contact, her subsequent therapy was uneventful.

Less widely appreciated are the other contraindications to observing the standard rules. The most common is the presence of a major mood disorder. Patients who have syndromal unipolar or bipolar depressions, even when these have been properly medicated, will almost certainly experience an exacerbation of symptoms in the relatively nonsupportive conditions imposed by the rules. No less important as a contraindication is the presence of borderline and other severe personality disorders. Patients who have dissociated saboteurs tend to engage in uncontrolled, destructive acting out if subjected to the frustrations of observing the rules. Such patients need, not neutrality and anonymity, but firm limits and warm caring to assuage the hurt and anger of their split-off parts. Only then can integration be expected to occur.

Other contraindications are extreme social isolation and value loss. Those who are chronically alone and without viable social networks cannot be expected to form interpersonal ties solely through an isolated, nondirective individual therapy. Group and family structures will usually have to be formed around them if they are to learn appropriate social roles. If the tendency toward relationship disruption is severe enough, the patient will have to be embedded in a therapeutic milieu to master the skills required to achieve stable intimate connections. Finally, demoralized patients who have no sustaining beliefs, who have lost the meaning of their lives and cannot find inspiring ideals, must not be expected to make good on these lacks with a blank-screen therapist who tries to assume a stance of moral neutrality. Rather, those who are disillusioned and morally bankrupt must find a therapist willing to serve as mentor—a personally concerned and trust-inspiring moral guide.

In summary, psychotherapy is a formalized relationship designed to relieve mental symptoms and to promote psychological growth. It is formalized in the sense that it follows certain rules (e.g., observing strict time and place boundaries and prohibiting physical contact between the participants) that run counter to the spirit of ordinary close relationships. The standard rules, which mainly derive from the psychodynamic school, have maturational, evocative, and teaching roles, but they should not be imposed unless their preconditions are met. These include the absence of major mood and psychotic disorders, acting-out personality disorder, social isolation, and value loss. When these are present, the other, nonpsychodynamic techniques of the bio-existential approach should be utilized to achieve optimal therapeutic outcomes.

I will now go over the specific rules in greater detail, moving from the rarely observed to the commonly espoused, in order to gain a better understanding of the indications for observing and abrogating them.

No Expectations of Positive Changes

For the therapist to disavow any interest in the patient's getting better he has to take an obviously paradoxical position. The usual reason is to disarm the passive-aggressive tendencies of those who would rather defeat parental-type authority, by rendering the therapist impotent, than get better. Of course, there are situations in which the odds are very poor for patients to achieve their stated goals, and it would be unwise for therapists to become too identified with these doubtful aims. No matter how much they think they want to, some clients are unlikely ever to get married or to achieve the status or wealth they seek, and making the success of therapy dependent on these outcomes is, to say the least, unwise. In such cases it may make sense to assume the classical psychodynamic position: It is the therapist's business only to provide insights, not to be overly concerned with the choices that patients make on account of them.

Yet in all other cases—that is, when patients are not intent on defeating the therapist and have a reasonable chance of achieving their stated goals—the therapist should get firmly behind them, affirming confidence in ultimate success. To do otherwise is to fall short of giving adequate support, in fact to risk coming off as the uncaring parent often encountered in the patient's childhood. For example, I expressed optimism about the prospects of an unmarried, middle-aged woman who desperately wanted to find a partner and was willing to work hard at it. Her narcissistic mother had repeatedly undermined her self-confidence by commenting unfavorably on her looks and dress. To combat these inner voices, I told her she would surely be married within a few years' time if she continued to work hard in therapy. Even though the actual prognosis for such an outcome was guarded, I knew I had to be unwavering in my expression of confidence in her ultimate success. Happily, three years later, she formed her first stable, reciprocal relationship with an appropriate man. Even though there has been no mention of marriage yet, she has become, perhaps for the first time, happy with the shape of her life. No harm, and surely some good, was done by my playing loosely with the facts of an unknowable future.

No First Names

By insisting on formal modes of address, the therapist seeks to affirm the professional rather than personal nature of the therapeutic relationship. This is certainly an important consideration in treating patients who are presumptuously overfamiliar or who refuse to take the work seriously. But in these less formal times, it no longer makes sense to fight the battle of professionalism on this terrain. Moreover, by leaving it up to the patient what to call the therapist, a valuable barometer of the patient's underlying attitudes is made available.

For example, a successful builder who was plagued with depression called me "Doctor" several times per minute in an excessively deferential tone. When this was pointed out, he began calling me by my first name and concurrently became increasingly nasty and disrespectful, so much so that the relationship was placed in jeopardy. When medicated better and questioned about his feelings, he began alternating between the two modes until he resolved the conflict. By not simply upholding the no-first-name rule, his therapy was provided with a clear window onto his hateful, ambivalent attitude toward parental authority—and also onto an important feature of his depressive disorder.

No Gifts

The danger posed to therapy by gifts is that they are inherently seductive and therefore potential levers of exploitation. By accepting a gift, the therapist may be coaxed into condoning some of the patient's faults and overlooking his or her acting out. By accepting a gift from the therapist, the patient may be cajoled into tolerating some of the therapist's acts of negligence. Clearly, the therapist has to keep a sharp eye out to prevent these corruptions of the therapeutic process. Doing so clears the way for a meaningful giving of gifts as an expression of genuine caring or as the vehicle of a holographic repair of core pathology, as in the case of Howard. Getting him to express a liking for a particular recording and then to accept it as a gift was the crucial step in overcoming his resistance to taking an antidepressant and subsequently overcoming his anorectic pathology.

An equally penetrating but quite different effect of a gift involved Carla, the lonely, divorced patient discussed in the last chapter who feared being poisoned by medication. Her psychotic mother was so poisonous that Carla regarded all gifts of food or medicine emanating from a parental figure as bad milk. After much reassurance and insight, she was finally able to swallow her antidepressant and let it work. She subsequently became much more open and friendly with me. To signal the greater warmth between us, I spontaneously gave her a flowerpot that she admired in my office. She was clearly very upset over taking it; a week later, she abruptly declared that she had gotten what she could from me and that she now wanted to be referred to a woman therapist.

I realized then that giving the gift had been sufficiently penetrating to expose Carla's core pathology. She had in fact dumped all the men in her life, including her father, ex-husband, and two prior therapists (as I will discuss further in Chapter 10). I decided not to interpret her behavior but rather to draw out the full implications of her having fired me: Although I would continue to monitor her medications if she wished, she could not stay on in group therapy with me, nor could she expect her ex-groupmates to continue to trust her. In fact, they dropped her as decisively as she had dropped me, and I did nothing to prevent it. Having now lost me and the group, she became suicidally depressed, reliving the abandonment feelings generated in childhood by having an unempathic, poisonous mother. All because I gave her a flowerpot!

The gift evoked the core paranoid response that had always disrupted her relationships with men and caused her to end up alone. Fortunately, I was then able to find the best possible reparative gift for her. Honoring her request for a woman therapist, I hooked her up with my colleague Mary Leshan, a very consistent, caring person with highly developed maternal qualities. In effect, I gave her the mother she never had; I also agreed to continue seeing her once a month for drug therapy.

With Mary's help, Carla worked through her abandonment depression. She set as her goal to get well enough to be able to return and finish her individual and group psychotherapy with me—in effect, to accept my gifts of caring without becoming rejecting or paranoid. Although in conventional terms the transference was split between two therapists, the split served to make good on a major deficit in her early mothering experiences. In a year's time, Carla sufficiently resolved her fear of being poisoned and penetrated by men to resume her therapy with me. Soon after returning, she became involved with the man that she went on to marry. It was her first lasting intimate romance. By violating the no-gift rule, I was able to uncover Carla's main relationship pathology for subsequent repair.

No Communications with Family or Friends

The privacy and confidentiality conferred by this rule are self-recommending. As the reader saw in Henry's case, bringing a spouse or parent into therapy can undermine the patient's efforts to get free of crippling influences from the past. Keeping the therapy scrupulously separate serves both a symbolic and real function in promoting the psychological separateness of the client. It can also help therapists resist competing claims made on their support so that they can remain unswervingly the patient's advocate. But there are situations in which these considerations are quite irrelevant, and even dangerous, to achieving a safe outcome. The following is a case in point.

Jean was an 18-year-old college freshman who was referred for depression and symptoms of anorexia nervosa. When first seen, she weighted 92 pounds, just short of appearing emaciated. Her mood improved on nortriptyline, but she was unable to gain meaningful insight into her self-destructive behavior. As the stresses of the college year mounted, her diet became ever more restricted until she was consuming only dressing-free salads and diet cola. Alarmed as her weight dipped into the mid 80s, I asked her parents to fly into town for a family conference, but they were unable to offer either insight or corrective influence. In fact, they had never been able to set effective limits on Jean's behavior.

Fortunately, her three college roommates came to the rescue. Concerned about her deteriorating condition, they asked to come to one of her therapy sessions. They offered to monitor Jean's diet and to put pressure on her to eat caloric foods. Even though Jean agreed to the plan, she soon had temper tantrums over their "interference." Once she began calling them obscene names, they realized that they had taken on more than they could handle. They were too preoccupied with Jean's condition to get their own schoolwork done. With my concurrence, they asked her to move out. Stung by the demotion of moving into a dingy room with a new, unwanted roommate, Jean started eating with a vengeance, rapidly regaining her normal weight of 115 pounds. By graduation 3 years later, she had become the manager of a successful restaurant!

Clearly, both family and friends had to be brought into Jean's therapy, because her life was in danger. Moreover, the individual therapy that respected her privacy had already proven inadequate to get her better. So serendipity orchestrated an outpatient form of milieu therapy that set effective limits on her anorectic behavior, at the cost of rudely violating her privacy. There are, of course, other situations when family and friends have to be brought into patients' therapy—for example, when they are incapable of caring for themselves or when they are too socially isolated to make independence a meaningful goal. Respecting the privacy rule is clearly antitherapeutic unless the patient is capable of exercising rational self-control.

Moral Neutrality

The severe personality disorders are characterized by *acting out,* a clinical term that implicitly points to the wrongness of behavior without emphasizing its moral valence. When we say that patients are acting out, we mean that their inconsiderate, exploitative, or dishonest mistreatment of others is motivated by psychological conflicts and effected by split-off parts of the self that are for the most part unconscious. We use this latter fact, the lack of conscious intent, to excuse the wrongdoer and to justify adopting the stance of moral neutrality. The advantages of this position are obvious: It is a humane, forgiving approach to human weakness, one that encourages nondefensive openness of communication and holds out hope for greater awareness and self-control in the future.

Yet there are clearly cases when therapists cannot and should not condone acting out, when they must take a strong stand against it. There are levels of exploitation and dangerousness that must be judged harshly and counteracted; adopting the stance of nonjudgmental neutrality in such cases might foster the perpetration of heinous, preventable crimes. In the face of an impending murder, there is at the very least a duty to invoke sources of restraint. Even in less dire circumstances, not taking a stand against destructive behavior would give patients little incentive to change and potential victims little chance to seek protection. The following is a case that raises some of these issues most strikingly.

Ralph was a 26-year-old office worker who came for treatment with vague depressive feelings, which I had difficulty pinning down. In the fourth month of once-a-week therapy, he told me how guilty he felt at age 10 when his 12-year-old brother, who had congenital heart disease, suddenly turned blue and died while they were roughhousing in a swimming pool. As he described this incident, he became frightened and shouted, "Oh no! Something is coming up that I don't want to talk about."

What he told me was that several years ago, after drinking in a bar with his girlfriend, he had driven her home in a torrential rainstorm. To his great shock, he saw too late that he was going to run over two people in a crosswalk. As he did so, he panicked and screamed, "Let's get out of here!" In a split second he became a criminal for life. The next day he read in the newspaper that the victims were a newly married couple, that the woman was dead and the man was in critical condition. He never looked at a newspaper again. About a week later he heard on the radio that the police had a suspect in custody. He stopped listening to the radio. It was now 6 years later, and he was depressed in my office.

In conventional therapy, the therapist would likely confine his efforts to exploring the reasons behind this gross piece of "acting out." Efforts would be made to uncover the patient's unconscious wishes and the relationship between his guilt over "killing" the older brother, committing this terrible hit-and-run, and becoming depressed. The hope would be that with understanding would come a measure of forgiveness and relief, and perhaps better control in the future. Out of a sense of what might be more helpful, however, I chose not to handle the case in the conventional way. Rather, I told Ralph that he had done a terrible thing, and that if he ever hoped to get undepressed again he would have to make amends for his behavior. I did not say what this would require, because I did not know; but amends would surely have to be made. Such an idea was, to my mind, the most important practical consequence of the existential-spiritual viewpoint: There was a moral ledger of objective values, and mental and physical health depended on restoring its balance.

With my support, he began the painful process of finding out the facts of the case—of determining who lived, who died, and who suffered for his crime. He discovered that the male victim recovered and remarried, but he could not bring himself to talk with the man directly. He also found out from reviewing old newspapers that the suspect was let go for insufficient evidence. After making these discoveries, he began to feel notably better. He was beginning the arduous process of balancing his books, the first step of which was to determine the size of the debt. It was, perhaps, not as large as he had feared.

With improved spirits, he came up with a reparative plan: He would seek training in a health care field. As a physiotherapist, he took great satisfaction in doing rehabilitative work. At the time of our last meeting, he was no longer significantly depressed. My sense was that my stern judgment of his immoral behavior, constituting an abrogation of the moral neutrality rule, had played a significant role in this outcome. Because Ralph had lost the meaning of his life, he needed a value transfusion. I felt that any treatment that hoped to be successful would have to restore his sense of moral worth and purpose. It could not afford to be "value free."

Anonymity

The anonymity rule is designed to remove the inhibiting role of the therapist's specific history and personality on the patient's capacity to project and transfer his or her feelings and primitive wishes into the treatment situation. Remaining anonymous and nondisclosing of their own attitudes, therapists become more evocative of the patients'. What is not often realized is that this is neither the only nor always the best way to evoke deep-seated wishes or reenactments. The same thing can be accomplished in group or family therapies in which the therapist is relatively forthcoming, for in these situations other patients, with their often greater similarity to significant figures from the patients' past, may serve as much more potent and natural evokers than the therapist could ever be. Thus, in the social therapies, the therapist can be highly present and self-disclosing with little loss of information because patients remain free to project unconscious feelings onto each other, which the therapist can then readily observe and help resolve.

Moreover, the inhibiting effect of therapist self-disclosure has been oversold. In many cases, nothing, least of all particulars of the therapist's history and attitudes, will stop the projection and transference processes. In fact, this is one of the main characteristics of borderline and other severe personality disorders; those who have them leak their underlying wishes and attitudes even in unfavorable circumstances. Having a self-disclosing therapist barely slows down the flow. In fact, "full-screen" therapists can be even more evocative than blank-screen ones. Because it is so rich and confusing, "telling all" and watching the play of responses can be extremely revealing, often unleashing in patients a flood of conscious and unconscious ideas. The corollary may also be true: Telling nothing often causes patients to clam up. And of the two strategies, the former provides clients with a fuller human being to identify with. These considerations become painfully evident in treating the children of blank-screen parents, as the following case illustrates.

Bruce was a 29-year-old physician; his case will be discussed further in Chapter 11. He suffered from intense generalized anxiety and inability to focus attention accompanied by racing thoughts, for which he underwent nondirective psychodynamic treatment for several years. In this therapy, no medications or cognitive-behavioral techniques had ever been tried. Instead, the impersonal therapist confined his interventions to scrutinizing Bruce's verbal associations for their unconscious content. Bruce found this quite helpful in allaying some of his anxieties and attention problems, but they would still burst forth and paralyze him every time he had to take an examination or became involved with a woman. Even so, he was grateful to his prior therapist for seeing him through the difficulties of getting into medical school.

Bruce's family history was notable for the fact that his mother had been in so-called psychoanalysis for more than 20 years. She was described as emotionally distant and scrupulously nondirective, a stance that masked well-honed skills at manipulating family members. In a caricature of the movie version of a therapist, she often deflected Bruce's questions with inquiries into his motives or surmises. Because of her guardedness, he knew very little about his grandparents or the details of his mother's early life with them. His father did little to counterbalance these trends. A passive man subtly dominated by his wife, he gave little guidance to Bruce, who characterized him as empty and ineffectual.

I intuitively grasped the meaning of Bruce's symptoms early on. Beyond biology, he was suffering the anxiety of feeling emotionally abandoned by his parents. Rather than more anonymity, he needed vigorous, empathic human contact. After bringing his anxiety symptoms under control with lithium therapy, I started my assault on parental anonymity. To test the waters, I moved from my regular chair to a place across from him on the couch. "You can't do that," he exclaimed. "Oh no?" I replied. "Why not?" "Because therapists don't just change chairs." As soon as he got comfortable with my nomadic ways, I told him that he worked too hard in therapy, that for the amount of money he was paying he ought to get me to do more of the talking. He thought this was both weird and refreshing.

Before long, he was asking me all about myself; I told him a great deal about my background and personal therapy. After a few weeks of listening to me, he began to get filled up. Then he started telling me about himself in earnest—his fears, his inadequacies, his hopes. When I put him in a group, he engaged in various forms of acting out, but he nondefensively took responsibility for his behavior. Most important, he expressed his anger toward his mother in his relationships with other women, whom he often seduced and then abandoned, expressing great shock at the hurt and anger that followed. Although the group came down hard on him for these activities, they also supported him in making changes. They became the warm, open family he had always wanted, and their discriminating advocacy helped him improve his performance in his residency and the quality of his close relationships.

By becoming a full-screen therapist, I had given Bruce more of a real relationship with me than conventional therapy usually affords. The justification for this was that he had never had a real relationship with his own parents. By bending the anonymity rule, his current therapy partially made good on this past deprivation.

But there are rules to this "game" of self-disclosure. Therapists cannot really "tell all" about themselves. They should not burden patients with current unsolved problems, only those they have brought to a successful conclusion. And they are foolish indeed to discuss the specifics of their intimate relationships or to stay in the mode of self-revelation beyond the patient's need for warm confidences. By adhering to these restrictions, some account of the therapist's own progress toward mental health can become a source of inspiration rather than apprehension.

Time and Place

Maintenance of time and place boundaries is crucial to fostering secondary as opposed to primary process thinking in patients. It helps them move away from a symbiotic merging with the therapist to an individuated mode of awareness. Insisting that patients come to the therapist's office at a specific time and for a specific duration is an ordering, responsibility-inducing requirement that sets clear limits on dependent clinging. Yet patients with borderline and psychotic disorders, most of whom have experienced severe early deprivation, may need to fuse temporarily with the therapist and be given "unlimited" care in order to make good on their personality deficits. Sometimes this may be effectively done by abrogating the time and place rules, as the following vignette illustrates.

My colleague Arlene Kramer, a naturally inventive therapist, came down with the flu and was unable to meet her office hours. She was very concerned about one of her clients, Emily, who had been abandoned by her mother in childhood and placed in a non-nurturant foster home. Once before when Arlene had canceled an appointment, Emily had become severely depressed and disorganized, failing to show up for work or her rescheduled sessions. Not wanting to repeat this experience, Arlene told her, in place of her office appointment, to come to her home and prepare lunch for her. Emily was surprisingly gratified at becoming a giver rather than receiver of care. She took pride in making a lavish lunch and a big fuss over Arlene's comfort.

Emily was clearly giving to Arlene the kind of care she wanted to receive from a mother while at the same time preserving Arlene's health and thereby preventing herself from being orphaned again. Although Arlene had always been generously nurturant to Emily, somehow reversing their roles and bringing her home turned the case around. From that point on, Emily began to make steady progress and eventually was able to become content with her life, an entirely unlikely prospect at the beginning of therapy. She dated her turnaround to "the time Arlene got sick." Most importantly, this was a one-time violation of the time and place rule. All subsequent sessions occurred in Arlene's office for the regular duration.

Fee-for-Service Payment

As I have already mentioned, setting a fee for therapy has both maturational and evocative effects. It forces patients to recognize the reciprocal nature of human relationships and to be responsible in "giving to get." If they enter into a fee-for-service contract and then have trouble paying in a timely fashion, then they either have fallen on hard times or are having psychological conflicts over dependency, retentiveness, or grandiosity, the standard grist for the therapy mill. By firmly insisting that clients pay up whether or not they fully understand the reasons for their resistance, therapists exert pressure toward greater psychological awareness and growth.

This approach, however, does not always work for borderline and other severe personality disorders. A strict enforcement of fee-for-service for these patients often stirs up destructive acting out that can derail the whole therapeutic process. To understand why this is so, we must remind ourselves that children are not expected to pay for parental care; they are entitled to receive it by virtue of being brought into the world. Though most therapy patients realize they are no longer children and cannot expect to be carried for free, borderlines have an angry, split-off child—an internal saboteur—that is still active and demands reparations. Because they have been traumatically shortchanged as children, they angrily resent having to pay for what should have come for free. Unless adjustments are made, then this part of the personality will experience therapy not as treatment but as more of the same old mistreatment that initially caused personality splitting. No less than with disadvantaged minorities, amends have to be made to borderlines for early deprivations.

How is this done? Clearly, therapists cannot usually lower their fees or give free sessions without devaluing their services and compromising their ability to earn a living. What they can do is give gifts, extra time, and other services, as I have shown in past case examples. One particularly effective method is to give free telephone time, often for the express purpose of monitoring drug therapy, but sometimes merely to assuage the patient's hurt feelings. A 2-minute weekend phone contact can see a severely disturbed borderline through a very painful "psychic bleed."

This was crucial to the success of Larry's treatment. Because he had been viciously abused by his father, he experienced intolerable episodes of rage as he became intimate with Linda. But with great reluctance, he was able to telephone during one of these episodes on a Sunday afternoon. Within a few minutes, I was able to soothe his feelings by giving him the consideration a good father should provide. He was astonished at how quickly and definitively this extra contact overcame his hurt and anger. This was one of several abrogations of the strict fee rule that helped Larry to subdue his angry-child saboteur.

As the reader has seen, giving actual presents can be a very complicated transaction. Both Howard and Carla had great difficulty accepting gifts. Yet in both instances, the evoked reactions were crucial to the favorable outcome of therapy.

Concluding Principles

The other rules against outside socializing and nondirectiveness are, of course, incompatible with the activist milieu approach I have illustrated in treating borderline patients who are otherwise incapable of sustaining intimacy. The effect of bending these rules has been amply illustrated by the many case examples given in prior chapters. Because I know of no convincing rationale for abrogating the "no sexual contact" rule and no clear-cut examples of its therapeutic benefits, I will bypass a discussion of this issue. What we must not bypass here are the principles of flexibility in observing and relaxing the standard rules.

The first principle is that therapists should learn how to apply the rules before taking liberties with them. This is accomplished by undergoing a rigorously supervised training program in which psychodynamic principles, as well as biological, cognitive-behavioral, and social approaches, are taught.

The second principle is that the rules should be observed to evoke symptoms, to strengthen patients' personal boundaries, and to foster individual initiative and responsibility. They should be relaxed to provide the symbiotic care and guidance that were massively lacking in some patients' early lives. In these deprived individuals, strictly enforcing the rules instills in therapy an element of cold formality and perfectionism.

The third principle is that the diagnostic indications for abrogating the rules are cases of psychosis, major mood disorder, severe character pathology, social isolation, and value loss. Everyday neurotics with intact social networks and value systems do not ordinarily require this kind of tampering.

The fourth principle is that broken rules should be reinstituted once the indications for breaking them are removed. When patients overcome their severe mood or personality disorders, then a good outcome may dictate that the therapist once again become more nondirective, anonymous, private, morally neutral, and bounded. Thus, breaking the rules is often only a temporary maneuver that is designed to promote a time-limited regression in the service of gaining subsequent self-development and integration.

SUMMARY

As a formalized relationship, psychotherapy must follow certain rules. In the standard psychodynamic treatment of neurotic patients, these include strictures concerning sexual contact, fees, time and place boundaries, focus of attention, nondirectiveness, privacy, confidentiality, outside socializing, physical contact, moral neutrality, anonymity, gifts, use of first names, and outcome expectations. Although following these rules tends to have evocative and maturational effects, they lie too far outside the capabilities and needs of nonneurotic patients, particularly those suffering from psychotic, major mood, and severe personality disorders. In these cases and in individuals with severe social isolation and value loss, a judicious relaxation has the effect of providing the warm, symbiotic care that is the birthright of children but that seriously ill adults have typically missed in their traumatic, split-inducing early lives. Yet abrogations of the rules should not be undertaken lightly. They should be the temporary fruits of extensive training and careful consideration. Once patients are capable of sustaining the forward maturational thrust fostered by observing the rules, then a more bounded approach should be reinstituted.

In this chapter, I have given several examples of a constructive, flexible alternation between observance and relaxation of rules in the service of first promoting a nurturant regression and then forward integration. In the next chapter, I will look more closely at the integrative process, particularly the specific means of overcoming dissociative splits in the personality.

NOTES

1. See the definition of psychotherapy in Chapter 2, which derives from Jerome Frank, *Persuasion and Healing*, Baltimore: Johns Hopkins Press, 1961.

CHAPTER 10

Reliving the Past or Creating the Future

Beyond symptom control, the major purpose of an intensive psychotherapy is to stop blindly reliving a destructive past; otherwise, there is no opportunity to create a productive future. The legacy of a traumatic early life is what all sufferers of major personality disorders have in common. Typically, they have all had a significant loss, devastating abuse, or narcissistic injury that threw them into a state of intolerable grief. For some, this overwhelming grief could be managed only by splitting off the suffering part of the personality from consciousness in order to numb the pain. It is this split-off, hurt, and angry self that forms the nucleus of internal saboteurs, which rob individuals of success in life by sabotaging their most cherished conscious plans.

Overcoming severe personality disorders involves healing the split that has produced the self-defeating hurt self. The initial reward for winning this struggle is the achievement of what Freud called *lieben* and *arbeiten,* that is, the attainment of deeply gratifying love relationships and a productive career. The ultimate payoffs, however, are bursts of creative achievement and enlightenment that come from opening a channel into the deep core of the self. The steps that are required to accomplish these elusive goals can now be examined. We must first look at the nature of the repressed or dissociated part and then the means of reclaiming it.

THE NATURE OF THE SPLIT-OFF PART

The split-off subpersonality typically takes the form of an *internal saboteur,* a private nemesis that causes mistakes and accidents that thwart the individual's most important aims. For example, Howard, who had for months come to his sessions on time and without mishap, took a wrong turn several blocks from my office and found himself on a back road miles away before he came to his senses. Prior to this mistake he was beginning to feel much closer to me, but his saboteur, taking exception to this development, led him astray. To avoid intimacy or productive confrontations, a saboteur will often cause the individual to miss the correct time or place of crucial appointments. Some potential clients are so ruled by their demons that they would never find their way to the therapist's office without special help, as in the case in which I had to flag down the patient's car outside my office. More ominously, saboteurs can provoke quite serious and even life-threatening accidents.

For example, Rick, whose father committed suicide at the onset of his adolescence, had major auto accidents the two times he became seriously involved with women. On the first occasion, after spending an intense weekend at his girlfriend's home, he awoke in a field next to the Blue Ridge Highway, having been miraculously thrown free of his totally demolished car. Two years later, Rick lost consciousness while crossing the Ben Franklin bridge and crashed into the protective railing. Once again, he was becoming emotionally involved with a young woman, a development that inspired another suicidal attack by his saboteur.

Similarly, a corporate headhunter who had been sexually molested by her father as a child, mysteriously began to botch her placements every time she began to enjoy some success at work. Another client broke his leg in freak accidents on three separate occasions, each time when he tried to establish some independence from his invasive, controlling mother who frequently gave him sexually arousing enemas as a child.

As mentioned before, perhaps the most significant saboteur in the annals of psychotherapy belonged to Freud. In his discussion of the fateful reliving of an unpleasant past, Freud in a veiled allusion to himself wrote, "Thus, we have come across people all of whose human relationships have the same outcome: such as the benefactor who is abandoned in anger after a time by each of his *protégés* . . . or the man whose friendships all end in betrayal by his friend."[1] Freud did not tell us if he was aware of the possibility that he was not simply the victim in the "betrayals" of Breuer, Fliess, Jung, Rank, Adler, and Stekel, but that the behavior of his own internal saboteur might have contributed to these repeated defections.

But is it really necessary to invoke such a notion? Is it not sufficient to speak of unconscious, self-destructive wishes or impulses? Certainly most theorists in the psychodynamic tradition have confined their interest to self-directed aggression as the major cause of self-defeat. Fairbairn (from an earlier generation) and Masterson (from current psychodynamic therapists) have been among the few who have accorded any importance to split-off saboteurs as etiological agents.[2] The reason they have done so is quite clear, if not widely accepted: The degree of intelligent planning, of ingenuity, that goes into most acts of self-sabotage far outstrips our ordinary notions of impulses or wishes.

Impulses do not ordinarily bide their time and wait for the person to drop his or her guard before attacking. They do not search out a boss's vulnerabilities before launching a provocation that gets the individual fired. But such finely judged maneuvers are the stock-in-trade of saboteurs. They are always on the lookout for timely opportunities to turn patients' victories into defeats, triumphs into tragedies. Moreover, they seem to have preferences for particular times, places, and modes of operating. In other words, whatever the wish content of their actions, they possess the added ingredient of personality style. Therefore, they are described better in terms of personal or quasi-personal agency than in the instinctual language of wishes, drives, and impulses.

Although self-destructiveness is the major currency of their business, dissociated subpersonalities also traffic in other commodities. These personal demons can function as sluts, whores, harsh judges, and even killers. One client, ordinarily a sedate, well-behaved religious woman named Lorraine, became a lewd, raucous temptress, whom she referred to as Linda, whenever she had a few drinks at a party. An auto mechanic under treatment for depression had, according to reliable witnesses, machine-gunned his own squadron mates in Vietnam. Suffering amnesia for the whole episode, he vehemently denied having done anything to merit his Section 8 discharge from the service. Whenever Amanda, a librarian of fundamentalist background, was overstressed at work, a voice inside viciously accused her of being evil and worthless; she referred to this archaic superego as "the Judge." She often began sessions by saying that the Judge had really been after her during the past week, that he had accused her of laziness and messing up on purpose, causing her to feel terrible about herself.

In all these cases of destructive subpersonalities, the object of psychotherapy is to gain conscious control of the split-off part and to integrate it with the mature observing self, so that the individual is no longer ruled by his or her unconscious but to some extent controls and channels it. For instance, as the Judge was reined in Amanda used its judging repertoire to prod her along the road of higher achievement. This paid off in her winning a management post at the library. The moderated judge then became a strict but motivating taskmaster for the employees that reported to her.

ELEMENTS OF THE SABOTEUR

But what goes into the formation of an internal saboteur? The school of transactional analysis points to the needy, vengeful child that persists in all adult neurotics. Quite clearly, other major characteristics derive from the patient's having identified with a depriving or injurious parent; we call this aspect of the saboteur a "bad introject." Yet other attributes fall into that limbo between biology and psychology that cannot be accounted for entirely by the conditions of the patient's upbringing. For example, therapists are surprised when they encounter overly scrupulous individuals who, it turns out, were raised quite permissively. In such cases suspicion arises as to the possibility of a strong biological predisposition to the behavior. And some saboteurs have such a strong ethnic flavor that one believes for the moment in a "racial unconscious," or such a murderous, suicidal rage that one flirts with the notion of a "death instinct." In the individual case, it is never entirely clear to what extent each of these factors—archaic child, bad introject, biological predisposition, destructive instinct, and racial unconscious—contributes to the distinct personality of the saboteur.

What is clear is that the view of unconscious processes being espoused here fits more comfortably with an ego or self psychology than an instinct or reflex theory. It assumes that what is repressed or split off is not just sexual, aggressive, or dependent needs but angry, libidinous, or needy "partial selves," who have not only dominant affects but characteristic mannerisms, instincts, reflexes, and cognitive styles. Of course, having such a partial self does not qualify the patient for a diagnosis of multiple personality disorder, which often involves the actions of several independent alter egos and disruptions in memory, identity, and consciousness. In the unstable personalities we are dealing with here, there is usually only one self-defeating part, typically activated by stress and accompanied only by minimal disturbances in the sense of self.0

Unfortunately, some therapists are so fascinated by the phenomena of dissociation that they encourage their more hysterical clients to bring out and amplify their partial selves into uncontrollable, destructive demons that cause personality disintegration. For example, a married artist, carelessly encouraged to bring out his gay self in an uncovering type of therapy, was soon engaged in compulsive homosexual cruising that jeopardized his health and broke up his family. Subpersonalities must not be encouraged to show themselves unless the means are already in place for limiting and reintegrating them into the mature healthy self. Integration, not further dissociation, is the aim of therapy.

REINTEGRATION

The reintegration of dissociated subpersonalities is an arduous task. In the simplest terms, the therapist has to activate the split-off, immature saboteur and then get it to rejoin the central personality, inducing it to once again cooperate in achieving the latter's goals. First, the saboteur must be exposed and reined in—grabbed by the throat, as it were, and prevented from blatantly acting out. Then the split is healed by inducing in the patient an altered state of consciousness in which *past grief and present relief exist side by side.* The grief derives from a reliving of the original loss or narcissistic injury, the precipitant of the early dissociation. In this state of reenacted pain, the correction and its healing relief must be simultaneously experienced. A "good enough" compensation or repair for the original loss or injury has to be provided. Only when the hurt self is so assuaged can it become responsive enough to be converted from a saboteur into an ally.

The following case histories illustrate how such corrective experiences are brought about. As will be apparent, reenacting the original grief often requires that the therapist behave in ways that are similar to the original mistreatment.

Carla

This 52-year-old divorced professional woman, mentioned in the last two chapters, was raised by a psychotically poisonous mother who withdrew her affection from Carla repeatedly and wrote her out of her will. Worse yet, when she did give approval, it was always done at the expense of Carla's sister ("You are so much smarter and prettier than she is"), so that their relationship was also poisoned. As a result, Carla developed paranoid fears about others' attempts to treat her well, particularly to feed or care for her. Moreover, in reenacting her pattern of escaping home by going from neighbor to neighbor, she went from man to man, dumping all the significant love interests in her life. As a result, she reached the midlife period all alone. Her calling card for therapy was, "I want to get married." After her fear of being poisoned by antidepressant medication was overcome, she felt better and much closer to me. As I indicated in the last chapter, I was moved to give her a flowerpot that she admired. Not surprisingly in retrospect, this brought out her intimacy-destroying saboteur, which demanded that she stop therapy with me and start with a woman therapist.

By this reaction, Carla provided a hologram of her failed love life: When she got close to a man and he was moved to give her affection, she responded to the gift as if she were being fed her mother's poisonous milk, provoking her to spit out the relationship. No longer going from man to man (or as she did earlier, from neighbor to neighbor), she now wanted to leave me and go to a woman therapist. The healthy current in this acting out was its cry for a nonpoisonous, good mother. Having exposed her saboteur, my job now was twofold: Definitively corral the saboteur, and then provide the corrective experience that would make good on her early mistreatment, thereby healing the personality split that arose out of it.

I accomplished the first task by making her pay dearly for dumping me—in effect, counterconditioning her distancing behavior. I withdrew my support and approval, and I passively allowed the loss of her group and the support of its members. Thus, in some ways, I was like her punitive mother. Yet there were important differences. I made her pay for good reasons rather than irrational ones, and I did it as a corrective experience rather than a vengeful punishment. Nevertheless, the losses seemed real enough that they precipitated in Carla an episode of intolerable grief, reminiscent of her early life traumas. At the same time, in her state of reenacted original grief, I was able to provide the needed corrective experience. I gave her the good mother, the woman therapist she had asked for, who nursed her through this perilous time by giving consistent, unambivalent caring and limits.

As she took in Mary Leshan's good mothering, Carla became less paranoid and more warmly receptive toward me. In her monthly medication visits, she became less fearful of being poisoned by antidepressants and more able to take in my suggestions without feeling violated. At the end of the year, she wound up her treatment with Mary and restarted her individual and group therapy with me. What group members noted most of all was that Carla had grown up: She no longer whined, and she took feedback to heart without becoming defensive. With me she was now openly affectionate and able to share some of her innate wisdom that had made her such an effective survivor.

The immediate payoff was greater career success. Carla enjoyed her work more and was rewarded with a substantial increase in income. Now she was ready to love a man without daring to dump him. Ted, a neighbor who had admired her from afar, at this point expressed interest in going out with her. Carla initially became frightened and had all her old borderline impulses to get rid of him. But by seeing her and Ted conjointly, I was able to help Carla lay her saboteur to final rest and heal the split in her personality. She lived through the courtship and embarked upon a happy marriage, as I shall discuss further in the next chapter.

Ben

This engineer first sought my help in his early 50s, after his wife of 15 years left him for another man. He was grief-stricken but manifested none of the vegetative signs of depression. Actually, the marriage had never been a happy one, and he was uncertain as to why he had entered into it. As far as I could determine, Ben had the dawning awareness that because he was still alone, in his late 30s, he was going to end up a lonely bachelor. When his wife-to-be showed interest in him at a party, he precipitously proposed to her after a very short courtship. No sooner were they married than he became moody and withdrawn, to her great distress. Though barely on speaking terms for much of the next few years, they nevertheless managed to have two children. But as the children grew older, silence grew into angry bickering over how they were to be raised. Ben had the overwhelming feeling that his wife was negligent in her care of them, and he resolved to show her how to do it right by becoming an obsessively perfectionist caretaker. As the situation became increasingly oppressive, she sought understanding and attention elsewhere, thereby precipitating his grief reaction.

I would never have understood the quality of Ben's upbringing had I not induced him to bring in his aging parents for a family session early on in treatment. It was not that he failed to tell me that his mother was anxious and paranoid and his father withdrawn and disapproving, but I had no sense of the magnitude of these character traits. In the flesh, his father was rigid like a board and totally devoid of affect, the closest thing to a lifeless robot that I had ever encountered in my practice. The mother, in contrast, was a quivering mass of jangled nerves, exclusively self-absorbed with endless paranoid fears. Neither parent knew what kind of work Ben did or who employed him. After the session, I realized that being fed, clothed, and agitated had been the full extent of his early care. As a child he had split off a schizoid saboteur to defend against the pain of failed intimacy with his parents; it was this distancing saboteur that would have to be corralled if he were ever to have a satisfactory love relationship.

To my astonishment, Ben physically flinched every time I expressed any feelings toward him. I was sorely tempted to retreat behind the screen of therapeutic neutrality, but two facts about him held out a glimmer of hope for higher goals. The first was that he had a good sense of humor;

he laughed readily and warmly, provided that emotional distance was maintained. The second was that he disliked his work because it was too impersonal and technician-like. He began to express regret that he had not himself become a doctor, because that had been his hope in college. He subsequently decided on engineering because the only faculty member who took a personal interest suggested that he would be suited for it.

Similarly, because I now took a definite interest in him, he decided to enroll in social work school to become a therapist. Although coming late to the field, he was able to earn a decent living, primarily doing hospital work. Just as important, he used his mental health education to understand the devastating impact of his childhood and to appreciate how sick his parents were.

Because he was socially isolated, I invited him to join a therapy group. Initially he related poorly to the other group members, finding it difficult to maintain eye contact or give feedback to others. He was attracted to Melanie, a divorced woman in the group, but his efforts to socialize with her were painfully inept. When they met for coffee or dinner after the group he talked endlessly about his work, unable to show interest in the specifics of her life. After a while, Melanie refused to spend time with him. Two years later, however, after he had worked diligently on his social skills and faced the fact of harboring a saboteur, he asked her out again. Although she was no longer in the group, Melanie still saw me occasionally for individual sessions, and I was able to put in a good word for Ben. Impressed with the progress he had made, she agreed to go out with him again.

Even though they now seemed to hit it off better, I realized that they would need guidance if they hoped to sustain their relationship. Ben was already in his late 50s, and Melanie was in her mid-40s; and even though both had been married and had children, neither had ever had an intimate love relationship before. On Ben's side, this was because he had a schizoid saboteur that destroyed the grounds for intimacy. At the slightest discomfort, he would suddenly become negative and critical and withdraw emotionally, which hurt Melanie's feelings deeply.

This negative, contact-avoiding saboteur had a devastating impact on Ben's clinical practice. After working hard to get clients into his office, he would drive them away by suddenly turning cold and nasty. Similar inconsistent behavior cast a pall on his therapy group; when he had to miss a group meeting, the other members were strikingly more spontaneous and interactive. Worst of all, when Melanie's children came home from college, Ben, after looking forward to their visits, made them feel like intruders by making hostile remarks. Because Melanie was a deeply devoted mother, Ben's behavior would have immediately doomed their relationship without my conciliatory efforts. Moreover, she easily became paranoid whenever Ben's saboteur created distance between them. Going beyond the facts of Ben's mistreatment, she developed the suspicion that I and her close friends were trying to make a fool of her. Fortunately, with the help of low-dose haloperidol, she could be helped beyond these painful feelings.

Having developed a close working relationship with both, I was now ready to try bonding them together, something comparable to introducing Linda into Larry's business, as discussed in Chapter 1. What I realized was that Ben, like a child, needed to be taken proper care of, something he had never experienced, and that not only was Melanie capable of doing it, she would in fact welcome the opportunity. Judging by her relationship to her children, who were warm and friendly, she was at her most effective in the role of mother. Her self-esteem was too low and she felt too easily penetrated and vulnerable to paranoia to tolerate a fully interactive partner. Also, her paranoid tendency to overcontrol was enough like his mother's personality to make Melanie deeply appealing to Ben, yet she was loving and responsive in all the important ways that his mother was not. Thus, with a strong intuitive sense of what would constitute a holographic corrective experience for Ben, I gave the following directive: Melanie was to be entirely in charge of their relationship, and Ben was to let her take complete care of him.

Initially they both thought I was joking, and they played along as if to humor me. After a while, however, they got caught up in the psychodrama of their prescribed behavior. In addition to entertaining him, telling stories and playing her guitar for him, Melanie drove him around and ordered for him in restaurants. In the process, Ben became more and more childlike. My expectation was that this present relief of past deprivation would reevoke the experience of past grief, but to my surprise this only came later. In the meanwhile, beyond using Melanie as an all-embracing mother, Ben was attentive to some of her needs and gave enough affection to make the exchange worthwhile for her. Even so, his fellow group members soon found the extent of his regression repugnant and prodded him to resume more adult behavior, which Melanie needed some help in adapting to. Within a few months, Melanie began to say what a wonderful guy Ben was: how kind and sensitive and totally unlike her former husband, who often berated her. She began to talk of being in love, which Ben found uncomfortable but tolerable. Then he began to let slip how much he appreciated Melanie, how warm and caring she was. And just as they began to achieve mutual love, Ben went into the long overdue period of grieving. He had periods of severe sadness and social withdrawal, interspersed with spells of great joy and happiness at having found Melanie.

In this state of split consciousness, additional antidepressant medication only seemed to intensify Ben's grief. As I have found in other similar cases, the medications seem to make the mature self undepressed enough to experience fully the deep depression of the hurt, childish part. As Ben went in and out of depression over the next several months, he spoke poignantly of the barrenness of his childhood, of the many times his mother and father violated his needs and hurt his feelings, which were attenuated only by splitting off a hurt, intimacy-destroying saboteur from consciousness. After his schizoid saboteur was assuaged—it was assigned the role of barring unwanted intruders into their private lives—Ben proposed to Melanie, and they embarked upon a marriage that, now 4 years along, has been remarkable for its harmony. Ben's occasional regressions into aloof sabotage have been managed by couples sessions.

Molly

This 44-year-old divorced research scientist sought help for anxiety and inability to make friends. As soon became apparent, however, she was plagued by a saboteur that hounded her to work all the time and that poisoned her lovemaking with anger. Shortly before seeing me, Molly had arranged to adopt Maria, a lively 6-year-old. Despairing of ever having another close relationship, she was prepared to settle for single parenthood. But no sooner had the adoption gone through than she met Evan, who quickly got very close to her and after a while asked her to move in with him. Somehow, adopting the child made Molly feel complete enough to entertain an adult relationship; yet having both Evan and Maria in her life was too much of a good thing. She began to feel intolerably unworthy of and exhausted by so much affection.

In truth, Molly was worn out by her saboteur's relentlessly lashing her to make work, not love. She had a full-time teaching position, numerous research grants to administer, a clinical training program, a child to care for, a mate to partner, and a household to run. As a lifelong workaholic, she was sleeping less than 5 hours a night and found herself bone tired at both ends of the day. She became irritable and disorganized and complained that she could not go on. Fearing that she might decompensate, I urged her (with group support) to take a month's sick leave, confining her activities to essential aspects of child care and tending to her research grants. She resisted the idea but was finally persuaded when she came down with a mononucleosis-like illness.

Resting at home, she entered an altered state of split awareness. On the one hand she slept late, read novels, listened to music, and joyously relaxed in a very uncharacteristic way. On the other hand, she was consumed with pain and guilt over not working. She remembered all the 16-hour workdays from childhood on her parents' farm. She recalled that if she or her sisters complained or misbehaved, they were spanked with two-by-fours. As a 6-year-old, she had 30 rabbits to feed and care of. It took her hours of exhausting work each day just to cut and gather the food for them.

As fury toward her parents began to surface, Molly tried to justify their behavior but became paralyzed by a mix of guilt and resentment. As a result, I suggested that she also take a vacation from seeing them until she worked through her feelings. At this point, she slipped on the ice and broke her foot; as a result, she looked more closely at her saboteur, which was apparently intent on not only making her work but punishing her for attempting to escape from the childhood conditioners of it. Painful as the injury was, it allowed Molly to prolong the sick leave and to steel herself against the saboteur. Only a short time later, however, she fell once again, this time injuring her back!

By the time she returned to her academic department, Molly had discovered that a great deal of her labor could either be delegated or dispensed with altogether. Moreover, she began to work out of genuine interest rather than fear and compulsion. She came up with research ideas that were more imaginative and potentially fruitful than her prior investigations. Then, in one of those tricks of fate that seem designed to further the aims of therapy, Molly was simultaneously elected to a highly prestigious national research council—marking her as one of the most promising scientists in her field—and notified by her department chairman that her contract might not be renewed after the current year and that she had to move to a smaller office.

The coincidence of being honored nationally and slighted at home brought another curative split. She associated the honor with being appreciated at her true worth by myself and her fellow group members and, in the past, by her teachers. The disparagement, in contrast, evoked memories of being beaten and treated by her parents as of she were nothing but slave labor. First she feared that she had been unmasked as the worthless person she had always suspected herself to be, but soon afterward she became furious at the department chairman for being so incompetent and insensitive, and at the institution for being such an "outhouse." Molly resolved to go out and find a better job, one more worthy of her talents. She relished the thought of confronting her chairman with his flagrant misjudgment and of leaving her unappreciative home. Fortunately, as soon as she took this stand, the chairman became more aware of her accomplishments and accorded her greater respect.

Before getting married, Molly had to resolve her sexual problem. Her saboteur would not allow her to enjoy lovemaking; if men came on to her, a part of her would feel physically abused and react with barely suppressed fury. Recognizing that her response was abnormal, she typically squelched her feelings and endured intercourse as an unpleasant duty, never able to achieve orgasm during the act. At a couples session, both Molly and Evan agreed, at my urging, to declare an indefinite moratorium on their sexual activities, concentrating instead on holding and comforting each other. This induced the necessary corrective experience. As Molly felt truly cared for in her own right, not as an exploited sex laborer, she began to feel intensely tender and receptive toward Evan. At the same time, she relived all the hurt and shame of the physical abuse—the beatings and forced work—that had characterized her childhood. Two weeks into the moratorium, Molly and Evan naturally slipped into intimate lovemaking, and for the first time she felt fully responsive and whole as a woman. After more than 40 years of feeling defective, Molly was free of her main hurts and splits, ready for the wedding that soon took place.

INDUCING THE CORRECTIVE SPLIT

The notion of a corrective emotional experience was Alexander and French's great contribution to psychotherapy. In their 1946 monograph *Psychoanalytic Therapy,* the authors argued for the importance of an emotional experience, not just intellectual insight, in overcoming the childhood psychogenesis of neurotic behavior.[3] As Alexander and French maintained, what corrected neurosis was being treated in the understanding mode of attuned parents rather than the rejecting mode of actual childhood, and being profoundly moved by the experienced disparity. Long before behavior and cognitive therapy were discovered, Alexander and French were espousing sound principles of cognitive-affective relearning.

Yet despite the obvious importance of the corrective emotional experience, the fact that it has not in subsequent decades been generally accepted as an essential ingredient of all successful, growth-producing therapy points to a problematic aspect of its clinical application. Alexander and French themselves discovered this very early when they tried to prescribe specifically corrective attitudes and responses among the staff of a psychiatric hospital ward and discovered that neither staff nor patients responded well. Beyond the adverse impact on treatment of prescribed, ungenuine behavior, the staff quickly discovered what all therapists everywhere have repeatedly discovered about people who have been mistreated in the past: They often resent being treated well in the present. Offering love to those who were not adequately loved as children, instead of making good on the deficit, very often adds to the feeling of being hurt and inadequate.

This is because the good treatment threatens the defenses that were originally erected against feeling unloved. In cases of only moderate deprivation, the invoked defense might be reaction formation, in which the person says, in effect, "I don't need your love," and makes a show of getting by without taking help and caring from others. But in the severe, traumatic deprivations that produce borderline and other acting-out personality disorders, the only defense adequate to the task of pain reduction is dissociative splitting, which yields a hurt, angry saboteur intent on alienating anyone who offers love in the present. The saboteur says, in effect, "Go to hell! I don't need your lousy love now. Where were you when I really needed you?"

Thus, by taking account of the phenomena of splitting and the formation of internal saboteurs, we are in a position to flesh out Alexander and French's concept of the corrective emotional experience. The previous discussion of corrective splits contains all the ingredients necessary to provide a model for overcoming personality disorders and achieving unity of the self. Not only must we give our clients the good parenting they never had as children, but we must be prepared to do battle with those parts of them that sabotage all such efforts. In explaining how this is done, I will first examine the preconditions and the nature of the therapeutic alliance; second, show how the angry saboteur is flushed out and its underlying depression exposed and treated; and third, explain how to heal the split and tame the saboteur.

THE THERAPEUTIC ALLIANCE

The sad fact is that along very important dimensions, we cannot help our clients do better than we have done ourselves. I do not mean that the single or gay therapist cannot sometimes help the blocked patient enter into a satisfactory heterosexual relationship, only that in many cases the limitations of therapists preclude their helping clients with similar limitations. This seems such an obvious point that one would not think it needs saying, but simple facts are often disregarded in our field. For

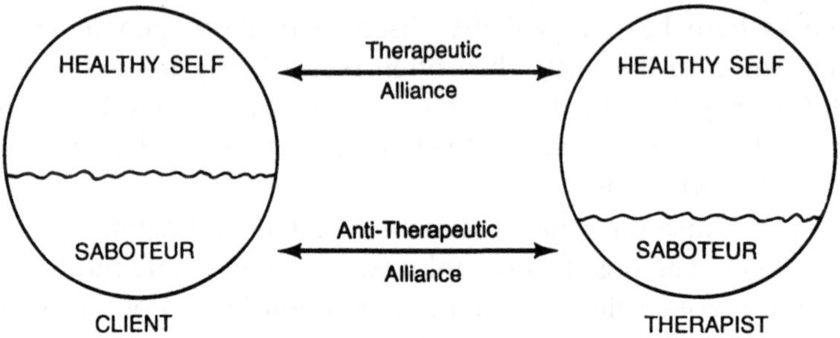

Figure 3. The therapist–client tetrad.

example, actively alcoholic or overeating counselors are not likely to help clients with these problems and ought not to try; those in masochistic relationships are rarely effective in helping others get out of such relationships.

We need a way of conceptualizing this nugget of clinical wisdom that both clarifies its meaning and furthers our understanding of splitting. The diagram in Figure 3 may help. In it we see that the patient and the therapist each have both an observing, healthy self and a split-off, sick self. For the sake of brevity, I have called the sick self a saboteur, even though it may sometimes function more as a killer, judge, or sleeze than as a saboteur.

The first point that has to be made is that for a patient to be capable of undergoing growth-producing therapy at all, the healthy self must be stronger than the saboteur; in business terms, it must have the controlling interest in the personality. This is indicated by the existence of "observing" ego and self-control, that is, the capacity to observe one's sick behavior as sick and to exercise the self-discipline needed to correct it. If, in contrast, the saboteur has gained majority control over the personality, then we say that the patient's will to health has been at least temporarily broken, as reflected in the clinical diagnoses of addiction, impulse disorder, or psychosis.

The second point is that for therapy to succeed, the therapist's mature self must be even more strongly in control of his or her personality (i.e., have more complete dominance over his or her own saboteur than the patient does). Otherwise, the patient's saboteur will have a fighting chance of thwarting all therapeutic progress by getting the therapist's saboteur to join in an unconscious antitherapeutic alliance devoted to fostering sick behavior. For instance, a therapist who took antidepressants for biological depression had many neurotic fears about taking her medication. She was very puzzled to see how many of her own clients for whom antidepressants had been prescribed also had problems with taking their medicine. According to her, she strongly encouraged them to take it as prescribed by the psychiatric consultant, but they were always forgetting or taking the wrong amount or getting into unusual problems with side effects. Only after she got more control of her own saboteur were her clients' problems with their medications quickly resolved. She had not realized that her saboteur had been unconsciously giving aid to the enemy.

Finally, a successful treatment outcome depends on the strength of the therapeutic alliance. This must be an alliance between the healthy self of the patient and the healthy self of the therapist, and the alliance must be stronger than the combined saboteurs' capacities to cause mischief. It must have strong enough elements of trust, affection, and respect to generate the loyalty that virtually precludes an untoward rupture. This is the greatest mischief that saboteurs can cause: to dissolve the therapeutic relationship for irrational reasons. When this occurs, the healthy self of the patient has caved in to the saboteur's unwarranted claims that the therapist has been so ineffective, wrong, or hurtful that the relationship should be terminated. To be sure, the therapist's saboteur sometimes plays a part in such outcomes by causing mistakes in treatment technique and preventing their correction. But in other cases, the therapeutic alliance simply fails the crucial test of being strong enough to counteract the regressive, destructive thrust of the client's saboteur.

How is such a strong bond formed? How do therapist and client make a connection that is resistent to the strong disruptive pressures typically encountered in the treatment of severe, acting-out personality disorders? For many years, students of psychotherapy have examined the so-called matching variables that make for strong therapeutic relationships: the qualities of understanding, empathy, and warmth on the therapist's part and the capacities for insight, self-control, and appreciation on the patient's. What is rarely mentioned in these discussions, however, is how important common interests and values are to the outcome. People who have similar tastes in art and humor, who are comparably moved by the moral beauty of certain actions, and who quickly reach tacit understandings with very few words exchanged are much more likely to form the strong therapeutic alliances needed to heal personality splits than therapists and clients who do not share a common mentality, who are not "birds of a feather."

EXPOSING THE SABOTEUR

There are two main ways to reveal a saboteur so that it may be neutralized: to observe it when it feels safely hidden, or to provoke it to show itself. The standard way to provoke an appearance is to prescribe behavior in the patient that threatens the saboteur and makes it protest. In the case of one patient, prescribing that he pay the family bills instead of his wife activated his greedy saboteur. If his wife had not been willing to report his behavior to me, however, the sabotage might have occurred outside the purview of therapy. Because neither of these possibilities—directing patients to act in certain ways, and getting family members or friends to report on their extra-therapy behavior—is permissible in traditional individual therapy, neutralizing saboteurs is not easily accomplished within the framework of its rules. But family, behavior, and milieu therapies address such issues quite comfortably, as the reader saw in the last chapter and in the historical review in Chapters 2 and 3. For example, the structural approach of Salvador Minuchin, with its emphasis on behavioral prescription within a family context, provokes saboteurs to reveal themselves and therefore is highly effective in correcting acting-out behavior.

To be lastingly effective with severe character flaws, the therapeutic approach must recognize the importance of splitting and saboteurs and have the tools to bring out the saboteurs and get them to become allies instead of enemies of the adult self. Getting the work done is a multistep procedure. The first step is always to begin working toward a strong therapeutic alliance; the second is to treat all mood and thought disorders with the appropriate biological agents. If the saboteur has not revealed itself by then, a behavioral prescription or an extra-therapy point of observation is instigated in order to "blow its cover." As the hurt, angry self is revealed, its raw feelings are assuaged by the "good enough" caring that it missed out on in childhood. In Molly's case, this involved being literally held instead of "fucked"—being valued in her own right, not for her performance. In Ben's case, being fully taken care of caused his hurt child belatedly to show itself.

Following the correction, the depression underlying the splitting defense is exposed; sufferers become profoundly grief-stricken over having had their boundless childhood love betrayed by inadequate parental care. Paradoxically, for many patients there is no possibility of exposing such grief unless its biological roots have been chemically pretreated, as the pain would simply be too great to endure. The mature self must itself be sufficiently protected from depression (by a favorable biological matrix and a strong, caring therapeutic alliance) to allow the hurt and angry child to relive its early, overwhelming grief. For healing to occur, the therapist must in the time of reexperienced grief provide the soothing, assuaging care, illuminated so well by Kohut and his followers,[4] that was terribly missed in childhood. In the process, the rebellious saboteur is induced to lay down its arms.

HEALING THE SPLIT AND TAMING THE SABOTEUR

Splitting occurs in the setting of intolerable grief. As the reader saw in Chapter 7, it is a radical defense that has the purpose of numbing overwhelming psychic pain and thereby preventing psychotic decompensation. The traumatized child splits off one small piece of the personality in order not to shatter it into many pieces, not one of which is strong enough to govern the self—the defining condition of psychosis. Because splitting is a numbing defense, the resulting split-off saboteur does its damage in the benumbed state. Patients engaged in major self-destructive or exploitative acting-out almost always feel numb about what they are doing. It is as though they are standing outside the action as an uninvolved observer, not as the enactor of the misdeeds.

This reported feeling of detached self-observation, of *la belle indifférence,* can first alert the therapist to the workings of a split-off subpersonality. Healing the split, therefore, involves overcoming the numbing defense and recapturing the original grief that brought it about. But because the grief initially was and still is intolerable, successful repair must safeguard the healthy, observing self from being shattered by pain. This is accomplished by building a strong therapeutic alliance in which the therapist can provide support and soothing and, where indicated, psychoactive medications that attenuate the level of distress.

What the therapist must provide within the therapeutic relationship—adequate biological and psychological care—is precisely what was not given to the patient as a child, thereby causing the traumatic grief that resulted in the formation of an internal saboteur. But as the reader has seen, the saboteur, instead of welcoming help, fights off all reparative efforts. Thus, healing is necessarily an aggressive, impositional feat that runs counter to the traditional rules of therapy and the training and temperament of many therapists, who understandably approach the treatment of patients having severe personality disorders with considerable misgivings.

But with the right approach (i.e., with the flexibility to alternate between being cautious and bold, and between adhering to and relaxing the rules), therapists can sometimes achieve success in healing the character flaws that lie at the heart of the major personality disorders. They can, in fact, help a selected group become reasonably integrated personalities. To do so, however, they must be willing to give (a) directives that provoke saboteurs to come out; (b) forceful limits (what I call "grabbing saboteurs by the throat") that prevent their acting-out; (c) accurately targeted support and caring that correct early deprivations; (d) medicines that attenuate mood and thought disorders; and (e) persuasive invitations for saboteurs to join the mature, healthy self. It is to this last point, how to recruit internal saboteurs, that I must now turn.

How does one convince a resentful saboteur to rejoin a self from which it had earlier defected? Certainly not just by pointing out the infantile, irrational character of its behavior—the sole interpretation that an earlier generation of therapists were taught to make. Both the positive and negative qualities of the saboteur have to be addressed, and both appreciation and firm limits (even penalties, as in Carla's case) have to be offered. On the positive side of the ledger, the split-off saboteur is often the repository of great strength and virtue, even a source of integrity (as it surely was in the case of Freud, whose saboteur did not allow for the compromises that might have forestalled the defections of some of his followers). Yet in many cases, the dissociation of the saboteur leaves the remainder of the personality seriously weakened. The normal funds of aggression, moral outrage, or sexual energy typically found in a healthy personality may have been depleted by its loss. Reclaiming the saboteur often leads to an immediate strengthening of character. For example, Cheryl, a depressed academic who later became an accomplished writer, experienced a "de-wimping" when she owned and made peace with her mean, hateful part. She began to express herself, in both her life and her work, with a rude vigor that was both exciting and effective. The case of Lucy, first encountered in Chapter 6, illustrates many of these points and gives some perspective on the proper balance between the cajoling and prodding that are required to heal serious character flaws.

Lucy

This 33-year-old attorney first sought psychotherapy when, after her sister became engaged, she realized she had become a workaholic with few prospects for a love life of her own. Most recently she had been in a 10-year sexual relationship with a man who would show up in the middle of the night to sleep with her but who never took her out on dates. Characterizing their relationship as "the longest one-night stand on record," she finally got fed up and told him she did not want to see him anymore. Apparently, though, she looked so bereft in the aftermath that her boss referred her for therapy.

Lucy was the youngest of three born to a dysfunctional coal-mining family. She remembered very little about her early life. What she did recall was that her father was drunk, abusive, and out of work throughout her childhood; as previously mentioned, she once drove him home from the neighborhood bar when she was 8. Her mother was a broken woman. Depressed and obese, her own father had told her, "You made your bed, and you will have to lie in it" when she complained about her husband's drinking and irresponsibility. Lucy came home at age 17 to find her mother lying dead on the floor while her father sat nearby in a chair, too drunk to call an ambulance. From that point on, she paid the mortgage on the family home out of her after-school earnings. To finance law school, she worked several jobs on the side. She and her sister spent all their spare money supporting the father in a nursing home, whereas their older brother declined to help out.

The history of Lucy's relationships revealed that she had a saboteur that forbade her to love an appropriate man. Because she was very pretty and a natural leader as a college student, several men fell in love with her and proposed marriage, but for reasons she did not fully understand, Lucy would dump them, often fixing them up with girlfriends. Yet men continued to ask her out until she began to wear thick glasses, dress poorly without makeup, and gain weight. She was 50 pounds overweight at the beginning of therapy. Apart from the long-running "one-night stand," she had not had a date in several years, and never a satisfying relationship with an equal partner. Despite looking depressed and suffering a narrowing of interests, she denied feeling depressed and was reluctant to admit she wanted a man in her life.

I was able to get Lucy to join a group to combat her compulsive overwork, but she initially resisted the group's feedback that she dressed and groomed poorly. Gradually her defenses relaxed, however, as we went over the dynamics of avoiding real partnerships with men. The parental model of a love relationship was repugnant to her, as was her mother's degraded, downtrodden role as wife. Moreover, she was already "married" to her sick father, and she had an internal saboteur that seemed intent on driving men away.

In the course of gaining understanding of her problems, Lucy became turned on by one of the group members. She asked why men like him did not ask her out. I told her without hesitation that a large part of it was her grooming and her weight. Greatly pained by my bluntness, she nevertheless resolved to make repairs. The very next session, she had a new hairdo, contact lenses, well-applied makeup, and stylish clothes; she said she had already joined a health club and lost 3 pounds. Her group was astonished at the transformation. Then men started asking her out, and colleagues commented on how well she looked. Lucy found it hard to believe that the few changes she made in her outward appearance would have such a profound social impact. But she had overlooked that outward changes often reflect inner ones, which others sense and react to.

She became more convinced that she had an internal saboteur when she ruined a budding relationship with a very eligible architect. He asked her out for a birthday celebration, something she looked forward to for days. On the big day, however, she went numb and shut down completely; she looked morose and could hardly carry on a conversation. He never called her again. When two subsequent relationships went sour for similar reasons, Lucy became clinically depressed, reexperiencing the grief of being repeatedly disappointed by her sick father and mother in childhood. After some arm-twisting, she agreed to take trazodone for her depressed feelings, and as it took effect, some of her childhood amnesia lifted. She recaptured many of the memories of the impact of her mother's depression and her father's fecklessness on her sense of confidence and security. This process was aided immeasurably by joint sessions with her older sister, who helped recall experiences Lucy had forgotten.

Gradually feeling stronger, she was able to look more searchingly at the structure of her relationships with men. On the one hand, she ruined every promising love relationship; on the other hand, she was ready to get involved with men who exploited her. This pattern had started with her father and brother and continued with her long "one-night stand," and she now found herself working for a boss who called her stupid and expected her to work 80 hours a week for beginner's wages. I decided that fixing Lucy's relationship with her boss, a father figure in her eyes, was our first priority because it would effect a holographic repair that would change her relationship to all important male figures.

I pushed Lucy to tell her boss to "knock it off" every time he spoke disrespectfully to her. Moreover, she was assigned the task of getting another job offer and then using it as leverage to demand a large pay increase and full partnership in her current firm. With my strong prodding, she accomplished every one of these goals within a few months' time and reaped the benefits of enhanced self-confidence and assertiveness. Although she complained that "therapy is much harder work than I ever imagined," she was now ready to fight the battle of finding a suitable partner.

As happened with Carla, a suitable partner turned up just as Lucy was about ready to have one. She attracted Doug's attention in church; on their first few dates, she was aware of both the strongest urge within her to scare him away and the grimmest determination not to let her saboteur get its way. She agreed to telephone me for a pep talk before she went out, particularly if she was aware of negative feelings about Doug. She complained that these dates were exhausting, because she had to watch her every move.

It was at this time that the episode described in Chapter 6 came about. When she was torn between driving up to take her father to the doctor and staying home in order to have time for Doug, I offered to drive up myself and transport her father to the doctor's office. By this offer, which of course I would have had to deliver on if asked, I undid her own parentification: I decisively became her parental caregiver and precluded her taking the parental role with her own father. To get her to accept that she must not continue to sacrifice her own life to care for him, I pointed out that she had been married to him and now had to divorce him. I also gave her credit for her basic loyalty and health; getting nothing in return, she had scrupulously obeyed the biblical commandment to honor her father. Her healthy self had so much wanted a proper father that she had propped up this shell of a man for more than 30 years. It was now time to have her own life and let other relatives look in on him.

Once she mastered her guilt over "abandoning" her father, Lucy developed increasing faith that she now had her saboteur by the throat. She maintained that she would never have had the energy and self-confidence to "divorce" her father and make herself available to Doug without the strengthening effects of the antidepressant medication and group support.

The first major test of this relationship came when Lucy was about to leave for a vacation that had been planned long before she met Doug. When he said he did not like the idea of her going away alone, Lucy took great offense, interpreting his remark as an attempt to control her. It took me some doing to convince her otherwise, that Doug was feeling protective and wanted to go along with her. Finally, she relented and admitted that a misunderstanding such as this in the past would have doomed the relationship.

Now that Lucy was getting her saboteur increasingly under control, she began the process of "reeling Doug in." When he declined to go to a party with her, she made plans without him the following weekend, which hurt his feelings and made him less ready to decline future invitations. When he asked her to sew a button on her shirt, she said she did not do such things for dates, only for boyfriends—a level of assertiveness impossible in her previously dissociated state. She was now ready to have a relationship in which she would settle for nothing less than equal partnership.

The reintegration of Lucy's internal saboteur was accomplished by helping her (a) become more vigilant of its relationship-destroying activities; (b) curb its acting-out by repeated acts of will; (c) assert herself toward male figures in ways that were incompatible with being mistreated and that expressed her true wishes; (d) "divorce" her father; and (e) admit to herself that she wanted a partner and would do what it took to form an intimate bond. The proof that the reintegration had occurred was an upsurge in her aggressiveness and her libido, which were now robust and constructive. Even though this relationship did not stand the test of time—Doug declined to seek help for his overinvolvement with his mother—Lucy was now ready to find the right person, with much less fear of sabotaging the connection.

SUMMARY AND CONCLUSIONS

In this chapter I have discussed some of the steps that must be taken to stop reliving the destructive behavior patterns that make up the severe personality disorders. Only then can individuals achieve the freedom to shape their present and future according to their own highest values. To support this understanding, I have explored the clinical phenomena of splitting and the resulting formation of an internal saboteur that acts out self-destructively. I have given numerous clinical examples of how splitting is overcome so that the saboteur is transformed into a constructive part of the personality.

The corrective repair of a split-off subpersonality involves inducing an altered state of consciousness in which past grief and current relief are simultaneously experienced. Assuaging the grief and depression underlying the early dissociation requires proper biological, psychological, and existential care. The existential part of this repair is the main subject of Chapter 12. It involves paying attention to what is often overlooked in psychotherapy: that the patient cannot overcome character flaws without reclaiming the creative self and finding a lifework.

NOTES

1. S. Freud, "Beyond the Pleasure Principle," in *Standard Edition*, vol. 18, p. 22.
2. W. R. D. Fairbairn, *Psychoanalytic Studies of the Personality*, London: Routledge and Kegan Paul, 1952; J. Masterson, *The Search for the Real Self*, New York: Free Press, 1988. Also see P. G. Vorhaus, "Spotting and Stopping the 'Inner Saboteur,' " *Psychoanalytic Review* 53:127–136, 1966.
3. F. Alexander and T. M. French, *Psychoanalytic Therapy*, New York: Ronald Press, 1946. Also see F. Alexander, *Psychoanalysis and Psychotherapy*, New York: W. W. Norton, 1956.
4. H. Kohut, *The Analysis of the Self*, New York: International Universities Press, 1971.

CHAPTER 11

Guided Intimacy and Milieu Therapy

As the reader has seen throughout this book, individuals with severe personality disorders have great difficulty in sustaining intimate relationships. Characteristically, they play host to internal saboteurs and other split-off subpersonalities that work at driving potential partners away. To overcome these "borderline" dynamics, I have devised a type of milieu therapy—illustrated by the cases of Beth and Howard and Melanie and Ben—that guides patients down the path of stable bond formation. In this approach the potential mates report on each other's intimacy-destroying behavior, both to me and to their group members. The latter also socialize with them outside of formal therapy time, report on their self-defeating behaviors, and give support for their caring, steadfast attention. This widens the scope of therapeutic observation and intervention, making it possible to generate enormous social pressure for patients to select only appropriate partners and then to connect closely with them.

I have now used this approach in 60 relationship pairs over a 10-year period of time. Of these, 13 have become romances and 8 have proceeded to stable marriages. (I plan to report on these pairings in a subsequent book.) The remaining 47 have been platonic friendships, of which 25 have become lastingly close. The vast majority of these individuals had not been able to sustain an intimate connection, according to criteria I shall later propose, prior to undergoing this form of therapy.

My purpose in this chapter is to describe the methods and the rationale I have devised for promoting stable bonds in unstable personalities. Because the traditional rules of therapy concerning directiveness, privacy, confidentiality, and outside socializing are abrogated by this approach, I want to first discuss the new rules that have been put in their place. Then I will address the definition of intimacy and the social repair of its disabilities.

THE RULES OF GUIDANCE

1. *When patients cannot meet partners on their own, the therapeutic milieu may introduce them.* Of course, it is preferable that people date as a result of natural, spontaneous extra-therapy attraction, as happened with Larry and Linda and Molly and Evan. But many borderlines cannot initiate relationships on their own, and almost certainly not with appropriate partners. In these cases the connecting may have to be done under therapeutic auspices. As with Beth and Howard, they may meet each other in a group and then be helped to get together, using therapeutic influence to overcome the forces of repulsion that arise between them. Because Beth was initially resistant to dating Howard, their relationship would have been aborted early without the added pressure and support afforded by the therapeutic situation.

This is even more the case when both parties are initially ambivalent. For example, Eva and Bruce, never-married members of the same group, gave little outward signs of mutual attraction. Even though Bruce (a 29-year-old medical resident with a bipolar disorder) said Eva (a 35-year-old professional woman who suffered from dysthymic and borderline symptoms) was too old for him, I sensed that they would be a good "practice" match, for they were both uncommonly perceptive and wise beyond their years. Not insignificantly, they had a similar kind of disowned, smoldering sensuality. Although they had had lovers and close friends before, these relationships had not worked out over time. One day at a group meeting, I suggested that since they were both currently alone, they ought to pal around together. Bruce diffidently agreed; Eva, oppositional and easily shamed, became incensed. Not only did she not want to go out with Bruce, but she accused me of betraying her trust by making the suggestion in public before asking her in private.

In truth, I had not sought her prior approval because I knew she was likely to veto the plan, against her own best interests. Only later did she admit that she had long harbored romantic fantasies about Bruce but was too proud to admit it; my suggestion had threatened to blow her cover of disinterest. Once she accused me of betraying her, however, I questioned the appropriateness of her staying in therapy with someone she regarded as a traitor. Realizing that she was skating on thin ice, she reversed her position and petulantly agreed to a date.

Eva and Bruce hit it off magically. Conversation flowed easily between them—the first hurdle of a successful match. Going to dinner and movies together, they started confiding in each other. Soon they almost slipped into having sex; but when they reported how hot and heavy it had gotten between them, the group reminded them of the rules of the milieu: dutch treat and no sex between group members. Knowing Bruce's tendency to become seductive and then run out on relationships, I interpreted his romantic ardor as acting out, setting Eva up for a big rejection that carried the freight of his hostility toward his undermining mother. With Eva, I warned her of getting in over her head. Prior to Bruce, she had scrupulously avoided having equal male partners; she only went out with "blue shirts" (as she called the construction workers and motorbikers she was attracted to), because she could run intellectual circles around them. She was afraid of Bruce, because he was a "white shirt." This admission allowed us to explore the quality of her low self-esteem and its dual origins in a biological mood disorder and a bad mother introject.

Eva and Bruce have developed a close platonic friendship that has set minimum standards for intimacy in any future relationship. It has given each a confidant with whom to discuss the most important life experiences, including dates with others. When they have reported on their outside contacts to the group, members for the most part have supported their relationship, taking them to task for any lapses in responsibility and kindness toward one another.

Two years later, they have remained each other's closest friend. Even though they had to be pushed together initially, they demonstrated a natural affinity. Seeing each of them separately has allowed me to influence them to resolve their differences when they have had misunderstandings or disagreements. Needless to say, any impulse to withdraw from this relationship as they had done in the past would expose them to a fair amount of social disapproval from me and their fellow group members. Although I have not seen them in couples sessions, I continue to see them together at weekly group meetings. Moreover, they see their group mates for meals and entertainment outside of sessions. It would be easy to overlook the crucial role this shared milieu has played in supporting their bond. In effect, they belong to the same team, and team loyalty must be served in how they treat each other.

2. *All guided relationships must initially be regarded as practice.* The treatment milieu cannot have a vested interest in any two people becoming

close friends, much less lovers or marital partners. For example, Beth and Carla respected each other but never got close. Yet they continued to give each other feedback in an attempt to remove the interpersonal debris that blocked their path to intimacy. Therapeutic goals are best served by regarding all connections between group members as practice for subsequent "real" intimacies. The reality is that, no matter how hard they try, some people do not connect. Moreover, a sizable proportion of these relationships will break up despite the support of the milieu. Therefore, it is best to discount this possibility from the beginning by regarding all milieu-supported connections not as ends in themselves but as rehearsals for subsequent friendships.

Thus, neither the therapist nor fellow patients can afford to become too closely identified with the goal of a consummated relationship. The major objective should always be new learning, no matter how close or distant the participants become. Otherwise, when milieu relationships capsize, therapy (to its great detriment) will be held responsible for aggravating the sense of interpersonal failure from which many of these patients already suffer greatly. Furthermore, having an overt or secret matchmaking agenda puts the sort of undue pressure on the partners that can call forth saboteurs to do their disruptive work. Yet, qualified, provisional milieu support still leaves the couple free subsequently to become real friends or lovers, and then to receive the backing they need to deepen and stabilize the bond.

3. *To form a stable relationship, unstable personalities need to be in conjoint individual (and, optimally, group) therapy, either with the same therapist or two therapists who are close collaborators.* Borderlines are notorious for stirring up antagonisms between different members of a treatment team. They externalize their internal splits. Two borderlines together can do more than twice as much damage as one, disrupting the relationship not only with each other but especially between different, potentially rivalrous therapists. Having a common therapist who supports bond formation is one way to circumvent the problem.

But such therapists, if they are to get away with this violation of the standard rules, must meet certain stringent criteria. They must be relatively resistant to borderline manipulativeness and countertransference hate,[1] and they must have tamed their competitive streak to the point that they are clearly impartial and even-handed. Most important of all, they must feel positive about the two people and their budding connection. They cannot, for instance, like one of them substantially more than the other. If these requirements cannot be met, then the therapist must bring a colleague into the picture, typically to treat the less favored partner. Ideally, this colleague should be a close coworker, one with whom there is mutual appreciation, open communication, and an absence of competitive envy. To take account of the various matching variables that different clients require, milieu therapists do well to have three or four such colleagues with different personality types in the circle of their work.

4. *Milieu members must get permission to date.* In order to meet outside, members must secure permission from the group as a whole, always with the therapist's advice and consent. To get this done, they must explain how the get-together stands to further their treatment goals. Thinking this through and winning permission cuts down on impulsive behavior. To minimize cliquish trends, beginning groups are encouraged to socialize en masse, not in pairs or threesomes; having a postmeeting luncheon or dinner together is a convenient format. Only with increasing maturity is it safe for members to go out in smaller subgroups.

5. *They must report on their get-togethers.* After permitted outside contacts, the participants are required to report on their experiences, telling the rest of the group what they did, how they got along, and what they noticed about each other's behavior. Differences in the reports of the participants and in the responses of the listeners are all fertile fields for therapeutic work. As mutual trust and familiarity grows, reporting can be allowed to become more implicit and informal. It must, of course, never be allowed to degenerate into tattling or gossip.

6. *No sexual or financial favors.* To preserve the independence and equality of each member, they are not allowed to pay for each other, have business or financial dealings, or have sexual contact. Each of these behaviors has the danger of creating an exploitation or collusion that works against the bond to the group as a whole. The clique that can result is the group equivalent of the internal saboteur, the manifestation of a group form of splitting that works against the overall goal of psychic integration.

The prohibition of sexual contact goes beyond the issue of clique formation. In our anything-goes society, premature physical intimacy is often used as a defense against psychological intimacy. Hopping into bed may be a way of short-circuiting the often painful process of getting to know each other, of sharing interests, fears, and vulnerabilities. Prohibiting it puts sex in its right place as something that one adds to friendship rather than uses to supplant it. As the reader saw in the case of Beth and Howard, their relationship had a long time to ripen before lovemaking entered into it. And even then, it had to be paid for by Beth's leaving the common group and struggling toward greater individuation. In short, the milieu approach discourages casual sex, certainly among borderlines. Rather, it advocates a responsible, carefully developed physical intimacy that comes to serve as a hologram of total psychological and spiritual intimacy.

7. *Patients appropriate for milieu guidance must be carefully selected.* Those who give a history of major difficulties in cooperating or in following rules should be excluded from such a vulnerable form of social therapy. By and large, individuals with significant psychopathic, addictive, and paranoid trends are unable to adhere firmly to social rule structures and therefore are likely to undermine the group cohesion and morale so vital to this process. The temptation to include them should be strongly resisted. Other selection factors include matching members as to severity of illness and basic values. In this program, one cannot include borderlines who frequently go over the border into psychosis, for managing their symptoms proves too distracting of the program's main focus on bond formation. Similarly, the program cannot accommodate individuals whose character flaws seriously interfere with honesty and steady commitment to the goals of milieu therapy. Another way of saying this is that only very high-functioning personality-disordered patients are appropriate for this approach.

8. *Patients who prove inappropriate must be promptly removed.* When failures in the selection process yield members who are persistently unable to adhere to the group's norms, they have to be promptly discharged. Whenever possible, this should be done as a temporary strategic retreat that serves to highlight the behavioral requirements of regaining membership; sometimes, though, the move is permanent. In the case of members who fall in love and want to sexualize their relationship, leaving the group is both an individuating separation and a celebration: a natural stage of growing maturity and independence. What usually happens in this situation is that only one member of the pair is required to leave. (This was the case with Beth and Howard, as described in Chapter 4.) Deciding which one usually forces an encounter concerning important issues of precedence and entitlement that had not previously been addressed by the couple.

9. *Outside socializing must be opened up to non-milieu members.* Outside socializing of fellow therapy patients needs frequent breaths of fresh air. It is very easy for groups to slip into cliquish and cultish ways in which

members feel they have all the answers and nothing better to talk about than their own therapy and therapists. To counteract these incestuous tendencies, outsiders must be included, and they must be treated with consideration (i.e., not made to feel like outsiders). This puts pressure on everyone to stay away from insider topics and from engaging in unbounded behaviors. By and large, all parties larger than four should include outsiders, as cultish tendencies tend to increase in proportion to group size.

10. Alternative therapies must be provided. Every group member should be in concurrent individual therapy, at least in the beginning phases of treatment. This provides a platform for processing the individual's group experiences: to assess feedback, uncover the origins of interpersonal conflicts, and set the goals of group and milieu therapy. Moreover, if the individual has to leave the group, the individual therapy can provide vital continuity of care. But, as I have discussed, the individual therapy relationship is no less vulnerable to borderline behavior than the group connection. Because it is the essence of the borderline condition to disrupt all relationships, individual as well as group, special steps must be taken to strengthen the overall bond to therapy.

One solution is to embed unstable personalities in a web of therapeutic relationships so that their primary individual and group connections are not their only therapeutic attachments. Thus, even though they succeed in severing some of the connecting strands, others can be put in place to provide a restraining net.

For example, Carla, the middle-aged professional woman discussed previously, dumped all the men in her life. Within a few years' time, she abandoned her father, her husband, a therapist, two lovers, and a professional mentor. Because I was certain to be next on the list, I saw her in concurrent individual, group, family, and drug therapy. When she came to fire me as her individual and group therapist, she had to first pay the consequences of her inconstancy by experiencing my disapproval and the banishment of her group members. Nevertheless, I made certain that she sustained contact with me as her drug therapist. I also referred her to a colleague, Mary Leshan, with whom I had a secure collaborative relationship that was relatively invulnerable to Carla's splitting maneuvers. Thus, I provided a holding therapy network that kept her close enough over time so that she could eventually bond with me and then a male partner.

First, Carla's lack of consistent mothering was made good on by Mary, who also pushed her to reevaluate her mistrust and disrespect toward me and, by extension, toward men in general. Once this was accomplished, Carla asked to return to individual and group therapy with me, having acknowledged Mary's contribution and respectfully taken leave of their individual relationship. Fortunately, Mary was my cotherapist in the group that Carla returned to, so that she could have the experience of having an intact, caring "family" to support her final move toward achieving a lasting intimate relationship.

Now strikingly more steadfast in our relationship, Carla fell in love with Ted, whom she referred to me for conjoint treatment. Thus, both she and Ted gave me the means to abort her subsequent (but now less vigorous) moves to disrupt the romance. And I could support Ted through the repeated small rejections that might otherwise have driven him away. The couple also socialized with other members of the milieu, who gave their blessings to the match and attended the wedding. Prior to this therapy, Carla had gone from age 40 to 50 without sustaining a single intimate love relationship. After their marriage, Carla and Ted gradually developed their own social network and became less involved with the therapeutic milieu.

The 10 rules of milieu guidance have been designed to make good on the abrogation of traditional therapy rules, particularly those prohibiting outside socializing and open reporting, which this approach entails. The new rules seek to ensure that group behavior is geared to the higher goal of achieving intimate human bonds by promoting a temporary, structured form of social enmeshment. At the same time they are meant to discourage the emergence of cultish, cliquish, and generally disruptive behaviors. Making certain that patients observe and report on mutual behavior and yet support each other for loyal and considerate caring are the primary goals of the rules of guidance. As soon as members achieve stable intimacy, they are encountered to form their own extra-therapy social networks and thereby gradually attenuate their connection to the treatment milieu.

Having described how intimate bonds are initiated and stabilized, we must now try to come up with the defining ingredients of intimacy and the rationale for employing the milieu approach when they are absent.

THE DEFINITION OF INTIMACY

According to our general understanding, intimate partners experience mental and physical attraction, express affection more than anger or disrespect, talk openly and spontaneously together, and have significant mutual interests, all on a consistent basis. When these qualities are significantly present, the partners take great pleasure in spending time together, typically sharing their common interests but sometimes pursuing separate activities. Thus, they are rarely at a loss for what to say or to do together, but in marked contrast to symbiotic partners, they respect each other's differences, allowing room for divergent interests and feelings. They also have mutual empathy, which involves taking pleasure in each other's happiness, and suffering through each other's losses.

When romance enters this picture of friendship, mutual interest extends into giving each other sensual and sexual pleasure. The partners learn to be comfortably naked and open together, to find enchantment in each other's physical being. The quality of their sexual intercourse becomes a hologram of their total psychological and spiritual connection. Thus, they know each other in both the biblical and psychic senses. Remarkably, they come to know what each other is thinking and feeling without having to be told. They are so empathically attuned as to be of one mind; for periods of time, they achieve a dual consciousness. But in contrast to symbiosis, the partners move in and out of these mental mergers to restore personal boundaries and interests.

As the reader has seen, patients with personality disorders cannot achieve intimacy on these terms. Because of mood and thought disorders and split-off subpersonalities, they are plagued by instabilities in both the initiation and maintenance of close relationships. From the outset, physical attraction for them is not a reliable guide to psychological fit. It is rather a dissociated yearning, often aimed at reliving an abusive or depriving formative relationship. Even when the attraction is mature, depressed and angry internal saboteurs may not allow the patient to enjoy the satisfactions afforded by the relationship. Moreover, in contrast to that for mature personalities, attraction for disordered patients is rarely an integrated response to the loved one's total mental, physical, and moral character. Therefore, because the different dimensions of the relationship are unevenly developed—sexy, perhaps, but not caring enough; highly respectful but less empathic—the partners do not work together in strengthening the bond, which is thereby rendered highly vulnerable to any disparity in their developing needs and interests. By contrast, when the different elements are balanced, the couple tends to keep pace with each other's life changes. They grow together instead of apart.

This analysis of failed intimacy quite clearly supports the therapist in launching biomedical, behavioral, psychodynamic, and existential interventions. It justifies medicating disruptive mood and thought disorders, deconditioning relationship-destroying habit patterns, defanging and integrating split-off antilibidinal saboteurs, and matching partners on the basis of common interests and values. But it fails to justify the program of milieu support that I have repeatedly described throughout this book. What is the rationale for embedding an unstable relationship in a supportive milieu? Why should this strengthen the bond between the partners? To come up with an answer, one must take a brief look at the social history of marriage.

THE PRIVATIZATION OF MARRIAGE

This is a time of unparalleled freedom for courting and selecting a mate. Without having to bother about anything or anyone else, men and woman can meet at public gatherings or through personal ads, feel mutual attraction, start to date, develop common interests and deep affection, and ultimately get married and start a family. Or, at any step along the way, they may change their minds and walk away. What is important is that the couple can make all decisions voluntarily and relatively free of external interference.

Of course, friends or families may try to fix couples up or break them apart, but these attempts lead more often to hard feelings than good outcomes. Typically regarded as meddling, they smack too much of the bad past when marriages were arranged. In past centuries, families and communities had a great deal to say about who courted and married. They made certain that considerations of property, wealth, and status operated in determining the suitability of matches. They even engaged professional matchmakers to get it right, to make certain that the respective families profited socially and materially from the resulting marriages.

What was often left out was how the individuals felt about each other. Did they like each other's looks, intelligence, sense of humor, personality, style, and system of values? Not enough attention was paid to these considerations. But as time passed and the world became more attuned to individuals' psychological as well as material needs, young people began to demand that their feelings be taken account of. No longer could mutual attraction and enjoyment be left out in favor of considerations of class and property. And the peer group, more cognizant of their friends' needs than the family or institutional authorities, began to play a larger role in fixing them up. Thus, after the period of arranged marriages came the period of social sponsorship, in which relatives and peers still brought couples together and supported their mating, but only if they expressed a liking for each other. Yet once the connection was made, the family and peer group continued to play an important role:

They monitored and influenced every stage of both the courtship and the marriage, holding the couple accountable to public standards of behavior. In other words, the family hadn't gone nuclear yet; it was still embedded in extended kinship and community networks.

But then the whole process spun out of social control. Edward Shorter, the great historian of the modern family, describes this evolution in very stark terms:

> At some point in the nineteenth century, the youth of Europe [and America] made a massive decision to withdraw courtship from collective control—and that means collective control of any kind. There is a kind of received sociological wisdom which says that courtship systems have passed from being community-run to being run by peer groups. But things didn't stop there. In the end, young men and women were no longer subject in their amorous lives to either the larger adult community or the subcommunity of their peers. Courtship had become privatized.[2]

This is exactly where things stand now. With respect to mating, young people are on their own. Accountability to family and society has gradually receded below the horizon of serious concern. By and large, men and women can marry whomever and whenever they want and, within the limits of legality, treat them as they please. If they do not choose to, they do not have to pay attention to social approval (who is there to give it?), ethnicity, geography, religion, social class, wealth, age, or even sexual orientation. They can make the choice of a mate exclusively a matter of immediate physical and mental liking. And the resulting families can live in anonymous privacy, far away from parents, grandparents, aunts, and uncles.

Of course, this creates its own problems. In the absence of outside matchmakers and stabilizers, only very strong personal attraction tends to bring people together. If the forces of attraction should be weak or blocked (as they were, for example, in the cases of Beth and Eva), then the individuals are unlikely to mate at all unless they are wealthy or beautiful enough to be regarded as trophies, or unless they find a social milieu that will guide their dating. Needless to say, these last conditions exist so rarely that the feared outcome of ending up alone becomes inevitable. It is a supreme irony that at a time when the freedom and desire to get married are at an all-time high, loneliness is the fate of so many who now lack an extended family to cushion the disappointment. The old social institutions for bringing them together—the schools, neighborhoods, church groups, and clubs—have withered on the vine of social change.

The second and more important problem is that this unbridled freedom of marital choice has contributed to an epidemic of marital breakup. As is well known, somewhere between one-third and one-half of all new marriages end in divorce. In exacerbation of the problem, couples are moving from city to city for better jobs. Increasingly cut off from the steadying influence of families, old friends, and the institutions of their upbringing, there are fewer and fewer restraints on jumping to new and better lovers, who are often (at least initially) more stimulating and less complaining than the old ones. Whereas in the past couples stayed together even if the flame of intimacy had gone out, old marriages now are being traded in like used cars.

Yet there is a good side to these developments. For many, the freedom of choice of modern times has brought with it a marked enhancement of the quality of relationships. Because of the fruits of psychotherapy and the dynamics of rapid cultural evolution, individuals are experiencing unparalleled psychological growth. And even though this sometimes entails outgrowing old mates, the opportunity exists to find new partners who are better able to share in the process of mutual growth and caring. Expectations have risen markedly as to what marriage should offer: not just physical care and pleasure, but emotional sustenance and spiritual attunement—in short, a continually deepening quality of intimacy.

Nor should we forget that more than 50% of newly married couples *do* stay together. Although some of these connections may be the products of encrusted habit or excessive regard for family feelings and finances, others represent successful intimacy on the highest terms. The couples have exercised their freedom first to fall in love and then to have their love grow in mutuality. From the start, they were integrated enough to be physically and mentally attracted to the right person. And they have stuck with their mates not just out of duty, but because their ability to communicate and to share interests and values has grown to ever-deepening levels of empathic caring. The bond between them has become solid and unbreakable.

What about the rest, for whom freedom has brought instability of relationships? Certainly a significant proportion suffer from unstable mood and personality disorders. For them, the withdrawal of courtship and marriage from collective control has served to expose underlying weaknesses of individual character structure; the withdrawal of external *splints* has uncovered internal *splits.* Different parts of the personality are not woven together into an integrated fabric of needs and values. Instead, warring subpersonalities swamp the self in a flood of ambivalent, rapidly betrayed commitments, so that discarded marital vows are only part of a widespread pattern of broken promises and lapses in loyalty. And there is no longer enough social glue to keep fragile personal connections from splitting apart in response to the buffeting.

As the reader has seen, medication, cognitive-behavior therapy, psychodynamic integration, and the realization of enhancing values are all vital components of a comprehensive program of repair. But if the analysis in this book is correct, a significant part of the problem derives not just from faulty biology and psychology but from miscarriages of social process. To overcome the resulting destabilization of relationships, a social remedy must also be sought. The historical process of privatizing courtship and romance may have to be, in selected cases, reversed. For those with severe personality disorders, who do not have the internal guidance and stability to make up for the surrounding social disintegration, mating may have to be returned to some arranged form of collective control. It may have to be subordinated to a system of community, family, and peer influences analogous to those that operated in past centuries.

As the reader can now better appreciate, this is exactly what the milieu guidance program tries to accomplish. In all the pairings I have discussed, courtship was embedded in a guiding social context. Couples were made accountable to a community of peers and parent surrogates, but on terms vastly more responsive to their psychological and spiritual needs than typically obtained in the past. The milieu programs foster a social regression in the service of ego bonding. What the 10 rules of guidance achieve is the formation of a peer group and a symbolic family that cares about the couple's need for love and that provides a noncultish matrix of support for initiating and deepening their intimate connections.

The milieu program, comprising conjoint forms of individual and group therapy, gives patients a social network to support the dating and mating processes. It influences them to select only appropriate partners and then to treat them with caring concern in order to achieve intimacy. Violations are met with both understanding and social disapproval. The power of these responses derives from the fact that milieu members are strongly committed to the group and care deeply about its feedback.

Why they care enough to be so powerfully affected is a matter of great interest. Before exploring the topic, we have to grant that well-integrated personalities do not require these external social pressures, because they carry them inside. They have internalized the words of caution and principles of value—sometimes reflecting quite conventional considerations of race and class—that caring families and friends have instilled in them since childhood. Consistent inner voices guide them toward appropriate matches and faithful caring. And they do not lack natural networks: close friends who double-date with them, give wedding showers, shop with them for homes and housewares, host their ceremonies, and see them off on their voyages of discovery. More often than not, however, patients with personality defects do not have these natural resources. Instead, they must develop them through special initiatives.

But this rarely comes easily. Many patients join athletic clubs or charitable organizations to make friends, but such steps do not usually lead to intimate partnerships. Even though they meet people there who share an interest, for example, in finding shelters for the homeless or building an arts complex, this common ground does not often provide a basis either for mutual liking or for sustained connections. What is missing? What does the therapeutic milieu provide that leads to successful matches (in our experience, more than half the time) that these ordinary social formats lack?

The crucial ingredient is a shared passionate commitment to a set of ultimate values. The therapeutic milieu engenders faith in a belief system that defines the main purposes of life—growth in awareness, psychic integrity, intimate love, and creative freedom—and the disciplined steps to achieving them. Finding a partner who shares in such a commitment is the strongest possible cement for a personal bond, given a base of mutual attraction. Common membership in an athletic club or a political organization does not provide such unifying higher ideals. Physical fitness and better government are certainly important values, but they are not bindingly universal in scope; they do not answer the call of the core of the personality for ultimate meaning. Achieving them together does not guarantee mutual personal fulfillment. In contrast, fervent, jointly committed attendance at a group program for psychological and spiritual growth (whose members are preselected for like-mindedness in this pursuit) inspires the kind of intense reverence and loyalty to higher ideals that binds individuals together.

When a group of people share a common belief in the main purposes of life and meet to work together toward achieving these ideals, then they develop a sense of *social communion.* This is the unique contribution of the milieu program to the therapeutic venture. Let us now look at the phenomenon more closely.

SOCIAL COMMUNION

As discussed in Chapter 2, Alfred Adler was the first depth psychologist to maintain that the search for social communion *(gemeinschaftsgefühl)* is an even more important dynamic in human motivation than sexual satisfaction. On this point he was irretrievably at odds with Freud, and hardly on the same wavelength with Jung and Rank. As often with Adler, however, his seemingly simple formulation reveals a profound truth.

To understand what is at stake here, we have to look at the definition of communion. It is variously described as

> a state marked by fellowship, sympathetic companionship, communication, and understanding . . . ; intimate, sympathetic, reverential, or mystic interchange of ideas and feelings, esp. dealing with matters innermost and spiritual in order to inspire, strengthen, or solace often as if between man and nature or the supernatural; a group of religious persons bound together by essential agreement in religious consciousness.[3]

Putting these various ideas together, I would say that social communion is a reverential exchange of ideas and feelings between fellow believers as to the ultimate purposes of therapy and life; the quality of the exchange and the nature of the sought-after ideals create a suprapersonal consciousness of spiritual intensity—call it *esprit de corps,* or heightened goodwill—that has inspirational properties for those who share in it.

Although I have not emphasized this aspect of the therapeutic milieu, it is perhaps its single most important quality. Newcomers are struck by the level of commitment and sense of reverence of the members for each other and the common task. As is true of all successful therapeutic groups, participants very soon begin to look forward with great expectation to the meetings. They cherish the sense of vital concern and understanding the members show toward each other. The group generates an inspiring, healing spirit that they yearn to connect with. They participate in a higher group consciousness that is dedicated to an unending growth in awareness and health that goes beyond the termination of therapy.

What is this group consciousness? It is an integration of several individual minds to create a larger group mind possessing intellectual and volitional powers that transcend those of the individual participants. On a smaller scale, intimacy between two people creates a dual consciousness, a merging of two minds into a combined single one. Embedding these potential dual minds in a larger web of consciousness generates powerful cohesive forces. Cohesion, no less than creativity or fanaticism, is one of the fundamental properties of mental aggregation. To appreciate this fact, one has only to watch flocks of birds and schools of fish move together as if guided by a common will. In human terms, these larger aggregations of consciousness produce supraindividual morale and will, profoundly unifying forces that have intrinsic bonding and healing properties. Anyone who comes in contact with such group spirit is automatically drawn into its vortex, which accounts for the strong yearning of the members to participate in it.

Set off against these integrative forces are the destructive possibilities of psychic fusion. As Gustave LeBon so clearly showed, these derive from uncontrolled chain reactions of the primitive aspects of mental aggregates, the lowest common denominator of the group. It causes group fervor to snowball into destructive fanaticism. Therefore, one of the major tasks of a milieu program is to generate the fervor while curtailing its potential for irrationality and intolerance. The system of control and accountability embodied in the rules of guidance is an effective means of achieving this goal.

Once one can ensure its safe channeling, how is integrative group fervor generated? To begin with, by careful patient selection. Patients with severe psychotic, paranoid, addictive, obsessive, and sociopathic trends do not tend to work constructively with any ideal-seeking group process. For the rest, it is important to match them as to basic values and drive to psychological growth. By and large, idealistic individuals work very poorly with materialistic ones; the dissatisfied, while inspired by success that starts far back and is hard won, have trouble making common cause with the self-satisfied. The guiding maxim is that birds of a feather not only flock together but become more united and creative once they do.

The personality and interests of therapists are also highly important, for these determine the power of their example and how they focus group discussion. Concerning the latter, they must above all steer the group away from incessant complaining about past mistreatment at the hands of parents, and they must dissuade group members from frequent exchanges of angry or hurt feelings. Although these are the stock-in-trade of traditional abreactive therapies (and remain important to overcoming emotional inhibitions in all modes of treatment), an exclusive preoccupation with them precludes the development of a higher group consciousness with inspirational properties. Instead, the group must stay focused on the main problems of psychological growth in everyday life: how to initiate, sustain, and deepen intimate relationships and meaningful work in the present. Past mistreatment comes into these discussions only long enough to understand the origins of inhibitions and self-defeating behavior, never to luxuriate in outrage.

Finally, for communion to occur, for groups to develop a fervor that binds people together and generates feats of creative achievement, the therapists themselves must exemplify higher ideals, both in the way they treat the group members and how they get them to treat each other. In their own presentations of self, they must be generous and ideal seeking, relatively disinterested in past or present resentment in favor of present enrichment. They must focus on the conditions of realizing intimate love and finding a creative, socially enriching lifework. The following case study illustrates how social communion was generated and how it helped a patient overcome social isolation and occupational drift to develop a rare quality of intimate, dual consciousness.

Cheryl

Cheryl, the college English teacher who became Beth's best friend (see Chapter 4), first entered treatment in her late 20s after her marriage broke up. After Cheryl met Timothy in the first year of college, they became inseparable as they took the same classes and worked toward their doctorates together. But their symbiotic fusion could not entirely conceal their submerged resentful and rivalrous feelings. When their first teaching posts required them to spend several days a week apart in neighboring cities, their common intellectual interests proved to be inadequate bonding forces. Timothy found a better position in the Midwest and disinvited Cheryl from joining him. She was crushed and became clinically depressed, weeping constantly and pining for her lost husband. She had virtually no friends to support her through the loss; in fact, she and Timothy had no social network outside their official connections to academia.

Referred by an acquaintance for therapy, Cheryl responded quickly to antidepressants and cognitive exercises. Her grief over the failed marriage diminished as she began to perceive its limitations and the forces that had led her to fuse with Timothy, a male version of her angry, hypercritical mother. Although her biological symptoms of depression cleared up within a few months of treatment, her social isolation and damaged drive toward intimacy took many years and all the resources of individual, group, and milieu therapy to heal.

Cheryl's sense of isolation had begun very early. Her Southern Catholic parents lived in a state of cold war. They rarely spoke, and they slept and ate in separate rooms. Cheryl was put in charge of her father, a warm but infantile alcoholic man. She greeted him at the door every evening and brought him his meals on trays, listening to his complaints about work. Her role of "daddy's girl" and oedipal victor had been established very early when her mother regularly put her in bed with her father while she herself slept in Cheryl's bed. This isolated, reclusive woman was phobic about germs: She avoided touching doorknobs and other people's dirty clothes, particularly those of her sons and husband, which she often kicked with her foot in disgust. Her mothering repertoire was confined to obsessive concern with diet, hygiene, and regular bowels. She finally separated from her husband after he retired and was home more often.

Cheryl was filled with bitterness about her mother's cold, angry, obsessive care, but her own life was permeated with its anhedonic, man-hating spirit, which deprived her of success in love and work. Whenever prosperity threatened to separate her life-style from her mother's, her saboteur would awaken and get her to quit or lose a job, or have another auto accident, or misplace her wallet (which happened there times in 2½ years!). She smashed up her car and went into major debt when, at my urging, she exchanged her shabby railroad flat for an attractive apartment on the Main Line. This upgrading move to better living conditions nevertheless served as a holographic repair of her impoverished life-style. After adapting to the improved circumstances, she began to dress more stylishly and to get better teaching jobs.

Getting Cheryl connected with a social network was the next priority. Isolated like her mother, she spent most weekends at home with her cat. When she first entered one of my groups, she felt overwhelmingly isolated, alien, and rejected. She tended to treat the gathering as a classroom where she competed for the teacher's approval. But slowly she won the members' affection and respect because of her intelligence, lively wit, and dedication to growth. At first offering insights that were too cutting or barbed, she gradually learned to tone down the academic critic in her and to bring out the enabling supporter. As a result, she began to connect, first with Ben (who was fatherly, and a fellow intellectual and loner) and then with Beth (her first close female friend, who helped her feel comfortable with being female and feminine). Beth taught her how to do her hair and makeup and to choose flattering clothes. In the process, Cheryl got caught up in the group spirit. In short, she had found a group of fellow workers who shared her fundamental values about psychological growth. She had found the caring family she never had.

Beth and other group members repeatedly tried to fix Cheryl up, but one date was all she needed to diagnose a candidate's deficiencies and scare him off. A first breakthrough came when she began dating two men she met at her health club. Even though neither one was judged to be adequate or acceptable, going back and forth between them kept her from focusing too strongly on either's faults. Moreover, having simultaneous affairs with two men was a major affront to her mother's and the church's code of behavior, and violating such taboos was liberating. I enjoined her to hold on to these two relationships at all costs. She complained but complied, calling them up when they failed to call her and keeping them flattered with her disowned Southern charms.

The second and decisive breakthrough came at Melanie and Ben's wedding. In the middle of the ceremony, she was overcome by jealousy, which she turned into a grim determination to end her isolation: "Goddamn it, if Ben can do it, so can I!" The very next weekend, Cheryl attended a concert with two group members, who tried to fix her up with one of their musician friends. But, difficult as always, she was disinterested in him but took a shine to his friend Jim, a successful professional man and amateur jazz player. They clicked right from the start. Jim was, in effect, a male version of Beth: manic, instinctive, and street-smart. For the first time, Cheryl returned from the first date—a Phillies baseball game, hardly in line with her usual highbrow tastes—without a single complaint or criticism. She and Jim shared a highly verbal intelligence, a deep love of music, and a taste for goofy humor and fun that had been masked in Cheryl by her hyperintellectuality. They took the time to become acquainted before becoming lovers. As they deepened their mutual respect and empathy, they fell deeply in love. They developed the kind of closeness that allowed them to know each other's thoughts and feelings without having to be told.

Although not critical of Jim, Cheryl could have easily been swayed to reject him if I or the group expressed disapproval. With trepidation, she introduced him to me, to Beth and Howard, and to Melanie and Ben. She needed to be repeatedly reassured that we all thought he was a wonderful catch. For the first time, Cheryl integrated her love life with her social life: She double-dated and partied with her group mates and friends rather than going guiltily on the sly, as she always had done in the past. Cheryl also connected to Jim's teenage daughter, who was desperately in need of consistent maternal care. Over the course of a year, Cheryl moved in, and the three of them formed a family together, sharing the meals Cheryl cooked for them with love and pride.

But the barriers to getting married would not fall spontaneously. On Cheryl's side, the problem was work. Dangerously close to getting everything she wanted from life, her love-hating saboteur acted out again and caused her to get laid off from her two most important teaching jobs. In a few short weeks, she managed to lose most of her sources of income.

The group was very concerned. Because many members had socialized with Jim, they (as well as Cheryl) knew he would be scared off by her inability to earn a living. Therefore, a part of her had to be trying to get rid of him. The group gave support and put pressure on her to make corrections, to combat this last hurrah of her mother-saboteur. Under the eye of group and individual therapy, Cheryl gradually put an end to the sabotage, got new jobs, and began to earn an adequate living again, without further relapses.

Jim had a very different kind of problem. Highly successful at work, he nullified his achievement by bad-mouthing his profession and guiltily giving away his potential savings to his still-undivorced first wife, Peggy, from whom he had been separated for more than 10 years. Cheryl succeeded in getting him to file for divorce. But despite their great domestic happiness, the months passed by, and Jim still could not bring himself to propose marriage. Actually, he could not afford it emotionally or financially, for he continued to pay Peggy large sums of support money, even though she was now remarried and there was no legal basis for doing so. A daunting fact was that many years of prior therapy had not resolved Jim's intimidated, being-taken-advantage-of connection to Peggy.

Now, feeling both internal and external pressure to put an end to this sick connection so that he could marry Cheryl, he began to have crippling panic attacks, which led him to seek me out for a consultation. I saw that he had a broad array of anxiety symptoms and masochistic behavior patterns. Although the symptoms improved markedly on fluoxetine, he was able to break out of his rut and set a wedding date only after intensive work in individual and group therapy.

Much like Cheryl, he became an ardent devotee of the treatment process, full of praise about the intellectual and moral values exemplified by the work and by my role in it. He soon achieved a sense of social communion that was almost as intense as hers. On this basis, he was able to look at the psychodynamic factors that prevented him from proposing. By paying Peggy, he was reenacting his masochistic attachment to his deceased mother, who always put pressure on him to satisfy her needs at the expense of his own creative impulses. He could not let go of Peggy because she was a stand-in for his draining, undermining mother, from whom he had emotionally cut off but never really separated. Also, by becoming happy with Cheryl and taking pleasure in his career success, he would be disloyal to the memory of his sadistic father, who had failed in business and marriage and died a broken man.

With this understanding, Jim gradually faced up to the unfairness to Cheryl of giving away so much of himself to past relationships.

Concurrently stopping the payments to Peggy, he was able to propose and set a wedding date. Cheryl and Jim got married in the garden at Beth and Howard's house. Melanie and Ben, myself, and other group members, along with the couple's increasingly numerous extra-therapy friends, were present at the ceremony and the reception that followed. The whole thing had a wonderful feel to it. Here were two people, surrounded by their close friends and associates, who loved each other greatly and who had worked hard together to create a deep and meaningful intimate relationship.

This case illustrates the role of social communion in overcoming the barriers to marriage of two patients with severe personality disorders. Embedding Cheryl and Jim in a network of colleagues committed to the same mode of treatment and the same high ideals of psychological development generated a sense of reverent commitment that, along with the other modes of treatment, overcame their intimacy-inhibiting behaviors. Neither patient had the kind of natural networks to overcome the centrifugal forces that had previously undermined their intimate connections. The treatment represented a rolling back of the clock to a time when marriages were sponsored by family and peer groups. But the surrogate family and peer network generated by milieu therapy has the striking advantage of being more biologically, psychologically, and existentially informed than any natural group is likely to be.

SUMMARY AND CONCLUSIONS

In this chapter, I have discussed some of the methods and values involved in generating an outpatient milieu strong enough to guide patients with unstable personalities into lasting intimate relationships. This involves all the techniques of the bio-existential approach, which is dedicated to overcoming mood and thought disorders, disruptive habit patterns, dissociated saboteurs, lost social networks, and deficient values. The outpatient milieu addresses the last two needs most directly. A successful deployment of the 10 rules of milieu guidance, by a therapist focused on present and future growth ideals rather than past resentments, is the best chance for deprivatizing courtship. It thereby places budding romances in a milieu with a strong enough sense of social communion to foster and cement intimate bonds, particularly in patients who on their own tend to disrupt them. To achieve a dual, intimate consciousness, the romantic pair is enmeshed in a group consciousness that generates strong cohesive, bonding forces.

NOTES

1. The topic of borderline and psychotic manipulativeness and its devastating impact on a hospital treatment team runs through my edited volume on hospital psychiatry; G. M. Abroms and N. S. Greenfield, *The New Hospital Psychiatry,* New York: Academic Press, 1971 (see Part 4, in particular). The discussion in J. T. Maltsberger and D. H. Buie, "Countertransference Hate in the Treatment of Suicidal Patients," *Arch Gen Psychiatry 30:*625–633, 1974, applies equally well to borderline patients who split the treatment team.
2. Edward Shorter, *The Making of the Modern Family,* New York: Basic Books, 1977, p. 159.
3. *Webster's Third New International Dictionary,* Springfield, MA: G. C. Merriam, 1966.

CHAPTER 12

Freedom

In the last chapter, I looked at methods for generating intimacy between partners and social communion among group members. In an intimate relationship, two individuals are able to merge their separate identities to form a dual consciousness of heightened empathic attunement. When this is done on healthy terms, the mergers occur in time-limited sequences that permit an intercurrent restitution of personal interests and boundaries. Similarly, when groups of individuals become close enough to achieve social communion, they develop a transiently shared group consciousness that has enhanced properties of cohesion and volition. As discussed in the last chapter, embedding a personal relationship, a budding dual consciousness, in such a group framework allows patients with unstable personalities to form the kind of lasting intimate bonds that they would otherwise disrupt.

What is striking about dual and group modes of consciousness is that they do far more than generate cohesive bonds among the participants. They also promote creative healing effects that are often striking and unexpected. Let us first look at some examples and then see what conclusions we can draw for the subject of creative freedom in general.

CREATIVE ACTS

The first case involves Barry, a married but socially isolated engineer who was referred to me by a colleague for group therapy after reaching an impasse in individual therapy. In his prior treatment, Barry had made excellent progress up to a point. Through medication and psychodynamic understanding, he had gotten over his long-standing depression, which started at age 9 when his father was killed in a farming accident.

But now at 42 he was stuck in a job he despised, working for a boss whose lack of support and appreciation reminded him of his stepfather's competitive undermining in adolescence. For the past few years, Barry had ruminated about starting his own engineering firm and being his own boss, but he could not bring himself to do it. He was unable either to find sufficient financial backing or to think of products that would sell in the marketplace. No infusions of support, insight, or medication could overcome Barry's paralysis or his social isolation.

Within a few weeks of the referral, however, he had connected strongly to his group and drawn on its will. He said he liked the members and their values. "They aren't bullshitters," he offered, "and they work hard at improving their lives." He greatly appreciated how positive they were about his plans to start his own firm and market worthwhile products. He was also impressed by how fulfilled many of them were in their own work. There was general agreement as to what things were worth doing, with psychological growth standing at the top of the list. It was clear that Barry had found a sense of communion with the group based on mutual appreciation and shared values. He had the feeling of belonging to a supportive family that worked hard and wanted him to be fulfilled in his life.

In this context, Barry quite unexpectedly stopped ruminating and came up with two marketable, socially useful products he could develop and be proud of, and he found a source of financial backing. With newfound drive and direction, he launched his business and, at the same time, became remarkably more animated and expressive. He began to make friends within the group and outside it, too. So far as I could determine, group membership was the only addition made to his competent prior individual therapy, the only factor that would account for his getting unstuck and coming alive.

Barry was freed up to become creative. Not only did he have new ideas about financing and products, but he now showed spontaneity in his interactions. Whereas previously his speech had been wooden, now he cracked jokes and made novel, insightful comments to his colleagues. Most importantly, group support enabled him to break out of a rut and start a lifework, a topic I will come back to shortly. This generated a level of excitement and enjoyment of life that he had not known since before his father's death.

The next case involves a more dramatic example of creative healing. Greta, 40 and too physically ill to work at her profession, had become utterly disillusioned at age 12 when she realized that her sick mother was only pretending to enjoy her piano playing, and was in fact not even listening. Overwhelmed with mortification—this was merely the crowning blow to a series of empathic failures—she felt something tear inside her and was overcome with nausea as she went numb. Although she was already an accomplished musician and graphic artist, she stopped drawing and playing the piano from that time on. Now, many years later and dying of systemic lupus, she overcame her amnesia for being physically abused during childhood by a sadistic maid. Rather than a saboteur, a self-hating, wishing-her-dead partial self had split off from consciousness at that time. Her lupus, a self-attacking disease, was a remarkably expressive physical analogue (a hologram, in effect) of these psychodynamics.

As the depression underlying these two dissociative experiences came into focus, Greta wept loudly, describing the past abuse and maternal neglect and expressing her self-hatred in almost unbearably explicit detail. Treated with the antidepressant fluoxetine and the full gamut of the bio-existential approach, she gradually overcame her dejected feelings. Moreover, she hungrily took in the support of her group, from which she made two close female friends. Encouraged by them to resume her art, she was at first resistant and full of excuses. But with encouragement from the milieu, she hesitantly began to draw again. Gradually, as I and her group responded to the results with appreciation, she went into a creative flow and began to paint oils and watercolors in a state of ecstasy. Whereas before she had experienced episodes of bitchy arrogance alternating with periods of self-loathing, now she poured all these feelings into her artwork, while she herself became more even tempered and satisfied. Her paintings, which she often brought to group meetings, were heaped with praise. With limits placed on her previously arrogant behavior, she began to treat her husband and children with greater consideration.

Greta's creative efforts were externally validated when she won two major art prizes. At about the same time, her lupus quite unexpectedly went into partial remission, and she entered upon a golden period of loving herself and enjoying her life. Greta had throttled her self-hating part, and she also reclaimed her creative self, with its artistic thrust, more than 30 years after first splitting them off. In the process she went into a creative flow and experienced a measure of psychosomatic healing. This way of conceiving the therapeutic result—as deriving in part from a reintegration of a defensively dissociated artistic self—obviously mirrors the prior discussions of reintegrating a split-off internal saboteur. Thus, the theory of dissociation, presented previously, has to be enlarged to accommodate not only saboteurs and guardians but more ecstatic, inventive parts of the personality.

The next case involves an upsurge of creative activity in a more explicitly religious mode. Cheryl, the English teacher discussed in the last chapter, described a childhood in which she was aware of an animate presence in nature. She felt that God, a more caring "parent" than her real ones could be, inhabited the forests and skies under which she played. She described her relationship to this living being as involving a kind of ecstatic, protective union that inspired flights of fantasy, prayer, and elaborate nature rituals. During adolescence, Cheryl lost this sense of connection; the trees and flowers went dead on her, becoming mere objects rather than living things. She recalls that the change took place while hearing a teacher deliver an incisive lecture on the difference between inductive and deductive logic. She saw clearly that the existence of God could not be proven by either. Suddenly her faith collapsed, and she became demoralized. Only many years later, after successful therapy, did Cheryl overcome the resulting sense of disillusionment.

There were three main steps to Cheryl's therapeutic progress. First, she had to get over her depression and make friends with Beth, Melanie and Ben, and other milieu members. Second and concurrently, she had to gain control over her saboteur, which was making her have accidents and undermining her successes. Third, she had to reclaim her spiritual self. The last came about quite dramatically.

Just prior to meeting Jim, Cheryl went on a camping trip with some friends. she woke up early in the morning and sat on a sand dune to watch the sun come up. As the sun's rays hit her face and chest, she had an illuminating, peak experience. She suddenly knew again that the world was alive and full of purpose and order, despite the rampant disorder visible everywhere. No longer was this awareness concretized in the image of a patriarchal God; rather, she directly perceived a mental organization in the cosmos that was the source of higher values. In this state of heightened sensibility, she was seized by the truth that her own mind was a cell in a larger tissue of consciousness informing the world. At the end of this experience, Cheryl knew that her life had irrevocably changed. Her childhood religiosity had been transformed into a mature form of spiritual understanding.

It was after this illuminating experience that Cheryl attended Melanie and Ben's wedding and became determined to find a mate. She visualized the outcome in intense, sharply focused meditations. In this striving frame of mind she met Jim, fell in love, and formed a close family. She also began to write fiction again, now with greater imagination and warmth than ever before. Instead of just grading papers and critiquing the writings of others, she had a burning desire to communicate her own perceptions and feelings. These arose out of a sense of being vitally connected to the cycles of birth and death, joy and suffering, and good and evil that constitute the world's natural order. Now less vulnerable to feeling either arrogant or worthless, she developed a steady, realistic sense of her own giftedness as a writer and human being.

In retrospect, Cheryl came to the realization that she had split off her aesthetic-creative-spiritual self, not just because of the limitations of logic but due to the emergence of her adolescent sexuality. In the face of her sex-hating mother and too-close father, she did not have the emotional support, the internal calming, to sustain both her sexuality and her spirituality on equal terms. She went into a state of painful conflict that had to be resolved. Rather than forfeit her sexual self, she split off the ecstatic, communing part of her personality, leaving her world a very dull, gray place throughout her entire young adulthood. She had become depressed in biological, psychodynamic, and existential terms. But her split-off creative self would periodically manifest itself as an arrogant, demanding subpersonality that was haughty and rejecting of her students, of colleagues, and above all of men who dared to come toward her. Her writings from this earlier period of her life tended to be overweening, empty displays of wit and virtuosity.

Once again, just as internal saboteurs get split off, so can the creative-spiritual self also become dissociated. Whereas the former most clearly occurs to attenuate intolerable feelings of depression, the latter also quiets the shame and humiliation of not being recognized as a special embodiment of beauty and truth. To understand better what she experienced when her spiritual self became dissociated, Cheryl, still the English professor, recommended that I reread Wordsworth's famous immortality ode. The following verses are most telling.[1]

Ode: Intimations of Immortality from Recollections of Early Childhood

There was a time when meadow, grove, and stream
The earth and every common sight,
To me did seem
Appareled in celestial light,
The glory and freshness of a dream.
It is not now as it hath been of yore—
Turn whereso'er I may,
By night or day,
The things which I have seen I now can see no more.

* * * * *

Our birth is but a sleep and a forgetting:
The Soul that rises with us
Hath had elsewhere its setting,
And cometh from afar:
Not in entire forgetfulness,
And not in utter nakedness,
But trailing clouds of glory do we come
From God, who is our home
Heaven lies about us in our infancy!
Shades of the prison-house begin to close
Upon the growing Boy
But he
Beholds the light, and whence it flows,
He sees it in his joy;
The Youth, who daily further from the east
Must travel, still is Nature's Priest.
And by the vision splendid
Is on his way attended;
At length the Man perceives it die away,
And fade into the light of common day.

Wordsworth seems to say that what is split off in early life is permanently lost to the adult, who is left only with intimations of the former splendor. He puts the attendant sense of resignation in the following mythic words:

What though the radiance which was once so bright
Be now forever taken from my sight
Though nothing can bring back the hour
Of splendor in the grass, of glory in the flower;
We will grieve not, rather find
Strength in what remains behind . . .

But the conclusion is needlessly pessimistic. Just as saboteurs can be reintegrated into the personality, so can the creative-spiritual self also be reclaimed. For Cheryl and others like her, the radiance was not taken forever from her sight; her "glory in the flower" was brought back, but now in adult terms. Of course, Wordsworth discusses these matters in the poetic-religious imagery of the soul's losing its connection with God. But the mission of a rational theory of psychotherapy is to recast such religious ideas, as much as possible, in psychological terms.

To accomplish this task, we can derive much help from Heinz Kohut's contributions to self psychology.

KOHUT AND THE GRANDIOSE SELF

In a stimulating series of publications beginning in the late 1960s,[2] Kohut struck a heavy blow against psychodynamic orthodoxy by showing that narcissistic grandiosity, far from being merely a defensive reaction in children, is a normal endowment that pursues its own independent line of development, separate from the instinctual drives and cognitive structures. In this way, Kohut called into question Freud's theory of infantile sexuality as the preeminent psychogenetic mechanism. No longer were the ordinary instincts to be regarded as the sole or even main motivating forces in human behavior and development; narcissism (or grandiosity) and its vicissitudes now assumed a central role.

According to Kohut, narcissism has two main channels of expression: the grandiose self and the idealized parental imago. In the former, the child feels full of self-importance and power, "the Lord of the Highchair." If empathic parents with high self-esteem respond to such a child with appreciation and "echoing approval" (perhaps what Rogers meant by "unconditional positive regard"), then the grandiosity is tamed into appropriate self-esteem and ambitious productivity. If, on the other hand, narcissistically injured parents fail to show empathic approval—or, worse, attempt to crack the narcissism by conveying that the child is "too big for his breeches"—then he or she becomes devastated with shame and humiliation. To attenuate the resulting pain, the grandiose self is split off.

In its dissociated, walled-off state, the grandiose self fails to mature with the rest of the personality and thus retains its primitive, archaic flavor into adulthood. It acts out under stress as a self-centered, obnoxiously conceited, coldly arrogant part of the personality; yet it suffers a "psychic bleed," a massively humiliating loss of self-esteem, whenever recognition and tribute are denied. Of course, if the grandiose self is very gifted, as in the case of a Wagner or a Nietzsche, it can produce valuable contributions to art and philosophy in its unintegrated state. On the other hand, if success and approbation are forthcoming, it may become overexcited and have to be shut down to curb painfully inflated feelings.

The grandiose self also searches for idealized parental models to revere and identify with. When the role models are adequate (i.e., when they personified good values and generate widespread respect), then they are worshipped as heroes and taken inside to become inspiring ego ideals. They provide personified belief systems that strengthen the will to produce and create. If the models fail, however, then the individual becomes disillusioned and demoralized and regresses into hypochondriacal self-preoccupation or enters on a hungry, never-ending quest for an external source of moral authority.

According to Kohut, having a split-off grandiose self and failed role model makes the individual into a narcissistically injured personality: self-centered, both arrogant and self-loathing, prone to shame and overexcitement, hungry for an outside god to worship, and acting out in typically narcissistic ways. By contrast, successful integration of the grandiose self and development of an effective belief system—what Kohut calls "idealization of the superego"—produce not only a mature person but one who has spiritual qualities: warmth, empathy, humor, wisdom, a well-grounded sense of worth, and above all, creativity inspired and channeled by good values.

What is very clear from this account is that Kohut, in characterizing the workings of the grandiose self, is describing the same part of the personality that I have been calling the creative or spiritual self. The grandiose self is the primitive, untamed, split-off form of the creative self. As the reader has seen, both Greta and Cheryl had elements of grandiosity mixed in with their artistic personalities, and taming these elements was vitally involved in reclaiming and disciplining their rich expressiveness. This also fits neatly with the discussion in Chapter 7 of the association between creativity and manic-depressive tendencies. What is perhaps less clear is that the grandiose-creative self is also related to what I have earlier referred to as the true self, the watchful guardian, or the guiding spirit. What all these conceptions have in common is that they refer to a part of the personality that has heightened powers of perception, moral-aesthetic judgment, and imaginative invention—manifestations of what Frederick Myers called the "subliminal" and Jung the "archetypal" self. Just as with the grandiose self, these parts of the personality can be pushed toward reintegration by a proper management of the mirroring and idealizing transferences that Kohut described.

This involves first an appreciative acceptance, rather than a reductive analysis, of the manifestations of the spiritual self. For example, when Cheryl described her religious illumination, I did not call it a psychotic episode or analyze its psychological mechanisms but rather praised the nobility of her vision. This was in marked contrast to her family's rejecting responses to her artistic and philosophical inclinations as a child. Subjected to ridicule and later to dissecting intellectual analysis, this highly creative part of her personality went into retreat, only later emboldened by therapy to come forward again. Similarly, Barry and Greta were given "echoing approval" for their inventions and creations. This enhanced their willingness to take further risks to develop their ideas and works, to show their creative private parts.

Secondly, the true grandiose self has to be harnessed to a set of justifying values and beliefs. It must be inspired by the high ideals of continuous psychological growth: of becoming increasingly more aware and effective, of undergoing an evolution of consciousness. The therapists and veteran patients encountered in the milieu come to personify these ideals. They provide examples of moral-aesthetic behavior that patients can identify with and emulate in finding their own ways to contribute. As Kohut has indicated, therapists and veteran patients must also be acknowledged for their advanced experience and achievements. In recognizing the moral authority of their mentors, grandiose, creative patients tame their high spirits and extravagant claims and channel them into constructive strivings.

As I have tried to show, I provided appreciative approval and generative role models in treating Barry, Greta, Cheryl, and many of the other patients discussed in this book. While attending to their depressions, bad habits, psychodynamic conflicts, and social deficiencies, I also used individual and group therapy to reclaim their creative parts. In bridging personality splits, these patients generated the power to express themselves in inventing, painting, writing, and philosophizing, all harnessed to actualizing beliefs and values that justified the effort.

But not everyone responds so effectively to these standard therapeutic techniques. Some patients do not so easily reclaim the spiritual self and become creative again. For them, additional hard work has to be done in the form of meditation.

MEDITATION AND THE CREATIVE SELF

For patients who have past histories of artistic activity or who experience periodic upsurges of creative flow, standard forms of psychotherapy (as conducted by an appreciative therapist who is also a generative role model) may catalyze the reintegration of the true self. But to make it a reliable contributor—and, even more, to invoke it for the first time—often requires the utilization of age-old methods of mental discipline, of which meditation and prayer are the best known. Techniques of meditation and their rationale have been expertly described by Herbert Benson[3] and by Lawrence LeShan.[4] Arthur Deikman[5] has performed the additional service of linking up psychotherapy with the broader subject of mystical thought, in which meditation plays a prominent role.

Exploring the topic makes clear that there are many ways to meditate. For each personality type, it is worth searching out the one or two most effective methods, a quest that may require the assistance of a therapist or guide who is adept in the field. For some it may involve a type of breathing exercise, for others a visualization technique, and yet for others a repetitive chanting or dancing. What is common to all is that they are mental disciplines and therefore highly analogous to physical disciplines. In fact, for moderns with a Western consciousness, successful meditation is best achieved in the context of a rigorous physical fitness program, of which it is a logical extension. Both are gymnastics: one of the body, the other of the soul. They both require a disciplined focusing of attention on a task that requires repetitive feats of effort.

A major part of the effort is to silence the voices of distraction and dissent, which try to dilute the individual's focused awareness. For at bottom, all meditations have as their goal one-pointed attention on the present task, whether it be jogging, eating, breathing, or making love. Of course, this is the hardest thing for a human being to achieve: to be completely into the present moment and the current task, with room neither for past losses nor future worries.

But as this is achieved, the greatest power that a person can know flows into his or her life: the heightening of consciousness that gives one access to the spiritual self. With it comes a dawning awareness of the infinite, universal mind that is the source of all wisdom and creativity. This is what Beethoven meant when he said, "I am not composing these symphonies; they are being composed through me." He had achieved a mode of consciousness that made him a conduit of a higher, universal will. What form of meditation he used to achieve inspiration, we do not know. He was perhaps so naturally focused and attuned that no specific measures were needed. By contrast, his fellow countryman, the philosopher Immanuel Kant, meditated by focusing his attention on a nearby church steeple for a period of time each day as he sat down to write his philosophical works. Thereby he cleared his mind of all distractions to the task at hand, which was to be inspired by a higher intelligence. Most importantly, he achieved this goal by pursuing a life of unparalleled discipline; his fellow citizens set their clocks by his comings and goings!

It is this issue of discipline that raises the greatest problem for those who would reclaim the creative self and thereby attain higher consciousness. Learning how to tune into the higher self presents much less of a problem than learning how to manage it once it flows into one's life. As the reader has seen, before the creative self is tamed, it is often afflicted with arrogance and grandiosity. Why is this so? Why is it inflated in its claims of power, knowledge, and worth? It is to this question that I now turn.

INFLATION AND THE CREATIVE SELF

It makes perfect sense that humans should be selfish and competitive. This is only fitting for territorial primates who sometimes need to protect themselves and do not always know when to stop. But what is there to be grandiose about? Are we just exhibitionists showing off our plumage, or is there something truly grand about us, however childish a form it sometimes takes? Although there are no final answers to such questions, it seems to me that grandiosity is a manifestation of a suprapersonal or transpersonal will operating in human affairs. What I mean is that the intuitive, creative part of the human mind has, as I have indicated, the capacity to tune into larger aggregates of consciousness than the merely personal. Functioning like a sensitive receiver, it taps into dual and group forms of mentality by attaining intimacy and social communion.

The most intuitively gifted among us, like Beethoven and other universal artists and spiritual leaders, have the capacity to commune with even larger aggregates of intelligence. Local heroes may have their fingers on the pulse of a regional consciousness, and national artists and leaders may serve as a conduit for a collective racial or ethnic unconscious. To the extent that they do so, we label them as charismatic leaders who have the gift of reading and directing the common will. At their most inspired, however, profoundly gifted individuals may draw on a supranational muse or creative spirit that transcends any narrow racial or nationalistic concerns to reach into the common soul of humanity. Because they reflect these universal modes of intelligence, the greatest scientific discoveries, works of art, and moral acts have universal appeal, finding as receptive an audience in Tokyo as in Tel Aviv.

But most importantly for our discussion, the possibility that the creative self can tap into ever larger aggregates of consciousness may explain why it can be suffused, in its untamed state, with a larger-than-life sense of ability and worth. It is reflecting the enhanced powers of knowing and willing that vast aggregates of consciousness would logically and inevitably possess. If these considerations are valid, the notion of the creative self is fleshed out to account for its proneness to grandiosity. I take this propensity as evidence that the spiritual self can intuitively connect to heightened, more universal modes of consciousness, with their attendant inflated moods and volitions. The immature, untamed manifestations of this connection are narcissistic, grandiose, exhibitionistic feelings. Its harnessed, productive forms involve a sense of creative flow that is permeated with feelings of ecstasy and truth. This sense of ecstatic fulfillment is the highest existential state of freedom, a condition of mind that gives new meaning to humankind's age-old search for a free will.

FREEDOM AND THE LIFEWORK

In one sense, the major impetus for writing this book has been to try to resolve the philosophical problem of freedom versus determinism. In its psychological aspect, the question becomes, how can humans be free to express themselves if so much of their behavior is unconsciously determined by their biological and psychological history? Posing such a problem is inescapable for therapists working with patients who cannot always escape the tyranny of their past lives but instead relive old self-defeating scenarios. At worst, they seem to be in the grip of a cruel fate, an external force dictating a life course gravely at odds with their conscious goals.

At the same time, modern psychological man knows, as Schopenhauer and Freud have taught us, that "we are ourselves bringing about what seems to be happening to us." We are the secret directors of our own tragedies. What we are now in a position to grasp is that the escape from this dilemma is to go beyond the determinism of individual psychology to become creative: to free our personal will by linking it up to a higher will. This commits the individual to enlarging his or her consciousness to a suprapersonal form and then drawing on its heightened powers of volition. We know this is being achieved in practical terms as the individual progressively falls in love with another person, with a group, and with a lifework.

A lifework is the spiritual opposite of having a job. A job has the connotation of following someone else's agenda, of painting "by the numbers." By contrast, a lifework involves drawing one's own pictures, expressing one's own innermost talents and vision. Such work comes from the true, creative self and therefore derives meaning from its capacity to connect to a larger, more universal intelligence. Thus, in addition to expressing the individual's best needs and talents—the ones most in need of fulfillment—it also taps into the aspirations of mankind as a whole, indeed of all living things. A lifework makes an altruistic contribution to the world while realizing the most important potentials of the individual human being.

Finding a lifework may come quite spontaneously, as it did with Barry, or it may be easily determined from a history of forfeited potential, as it was with Greta and Cheryl. But in other cases, it may require the most refined skills of the existential therapist, who is able to read fantasies, dreams, and behavioral leaks for their holographic significance (i.e., for what they reveal about the individual's core yearnings). It may also commit the individual to countless hours of solitude devoted to a rigorous program of physical and mental conditioning, of which meditation is a crucial component. Hard as it may be to do, there is no mistaking when a lifework has been found, for pursuing it suffuses the person's life with creative ecstasy and a heightened sense of meaning. In Maslow's sense, the individual enjoys a series of peak experiences in which there is a fusion of facts and values,[6] in which the most directly perceived facts are intuitions of value.

For natural artists, this may come about effortlessly and unconsciously, without the help of therapy. But for patients whose creative expression has been blocked by character problems, a broad-gauged, multidimensional treatment (sometimes supplemented by physical and mental meditations) will usually be required to free and direct the creative will. One or more of the following steps of the bio-existential hierarchy of treatment are crucial to success.

1. The correction of bad biology, particularly retarded depression, which blocks the spontaneous flow of feelings and thoughts. Also important is to conquer the kind of disorganization and paranoia that makes us react to imagined fears and irrelevant directives instead of our own best interests.
2. Overcoming past conditioning, particularly the kind that has resulted in learned helplessness rather than the optimistic taking of initiative, but also old indoctrinations that promote rigid, dogmatic thinking.
3. Subduing and integrating internal saboteurs and other partial selves with hidden destructive agendas that defeat the conscious aims of the true self.

4. Overcoming social isolation, not at the expense of necessary periods of solitude, but to enhance the individual will by unifying it with dual and group forms of consciousness. When the individual joins up with another person in an intimate relationship and with a group in social communion, the single mind is strengthened by collective forces of bonding, awareness, and volition. The enormous infusion of group spirit expands the power of the individual will and confers on it an empirical sense of freedom.
5. Developing a belief system that paves the way to higher consciousness. For the therapy patient, none is more effective than a self-fulfilling commitment to the value of continuous psychological growth. A final stage of this developmental process is the reclamation of the creative-spiritual self from its dissociated state by a proper management of the mirroring and idealizing transferences. But such efforts may not be successful without going beyond psychology into meditation and prayer.

Because the creative self has heightened intuitive capacities, it can from time to time tune into universal modes of awareness. At these moments, the individual achieves larger-than-life powers of volition and their accompanying feelings of ecstatic grandeur. To obviate the risk of spoiling such an achievement by the creeping in of narcissistic grandiosity, nothing is more important at such times than to have a rigorous mental and physical discipline, involving not only meditation but such other regimens as a daily work schedule and a strenuous exercise program.

In pursuing this demanding life course, the individual should ideally have both a personal guide, typically in the form of a therapist, and an intimate love partner. Both are needed to provide the necessary support and stability for an undertaking so vulnerable to miscarriage. In their absence, doing the work of reclaiming the higher self often leads to fanaticisms and compulsions that distort both the ends and the means of the process. Tuning into the spiritual self on appropriately stringent terms, in marked contrast, tenders the gift of existential freedom, the crowning achievement in the quest for human liberty. It is recognized by the experience of ecstatic fulfillment that accompanies its free expression in pursuing a lifework.

By ascending the bio-existential hierarchy and throwing off the shackles placed on the individual will at the biological, behavioral, psychodynamic, social, and existential levels, suffering human beings become free on all the planes of their existence. They achieve biological, psychological, and spiritual health.

SUMMARY AND CONCLUSIONS

In this last chapter, I have explored the possibility of gaining access to the creative self, of reclaiming the split-off artistic subpersonality. I have argued that this partial self is dissociated in early development in much the same way and for many of the same reasons that internal saboteurs are split off: to ward off feelings of depression, shame, and emotional flooding. In either case, the personality has to be unified from within and without. First, the individual has to reclaim all split-off partial selves to form a unified, cohesive individual self. Then he or she has to unite with other individuals to achieve intimate relationships and with groups to achieve social communion. The dual and group modes of awareness that result, which involve going beyond a personal to a suprapersonal mode of consciousness, have enhanced cohesive and healing properties that represent enlargement of the individual's love and will.

To go beyond these dual and small group aggregates of consciousness, often with the help of meditative practices, and to tap into a universal mode of awareness is the crowning glory of human freedom. By ascending the bio-existential hierarchy, we can progressively remove the biological, behavioral, psychodynamic, and social barriers to creative expression. The richest fruit is the practice of a lifework that fills our days with rapturous joy. We fulfill ourselves, and we make a contribution to humankind. This is the true freedom of the self.

NOTES

1. William Wordsworth, "Ode: Intimations of Immortality from Recollections of Early Childhood," in *Norton Anthology of Poetry*, 3rd ed., New York: W. W. Norton, 1983, pp. 551–555 [original date of poem—1806].
2. H. Kohut, "The Psychoanalytic Treatment of Narcissistic Personality Disorders," *Psychoanalytic Study of the Child* 23:86–113, 1968; idem, *The Analysis of the Self*, New York: International Universities Press, 1971; idem, *The Restoration of the Self*, New York: International Universities Press, 1977. Also see P. H. Ornstein, "On Narcissism: Beyond the Introduction," *Annals of Psychoanalysis* 55:241–247, 1974.
3. H. Benson, *The Relaxation Response*, New York: Avon Books, 1976.
4. L. LeShan, *How to Meditate*, New York: Bantam Books, 1975.
5. A. J. Deikman, *The Observing Self*, Boston: Beacon Press, 1982.
6. A. H. Maslow, *The Farther Reaches of Human Nature*, New York: Viking Press, 1971.

Index

MIX
Papier aus verantwortungsvollen Quellen
Paper from responsible sources
FSC® C105338

If you have any concerns about our products,
you can contact us on
ProductSafety@springernature.com

In case Publisher is established outside the EU,
the EU authorized representative is:
Springer Nature Customer Service Center GmbH
Europaplatz 3, 69115 Heidelberg, Germany

Printed by Libri Plureos GmbH
in Hamburg, Germany